THE VALUE BASE OF SOCIAL WORK AND SOCIAL CARE

THE VALUE BASE OF SOCIAL WORK AND SOCIAL CARE

Edited by Adam Barnard, Nigel Horner and Jim Wild

 Open University Press

Open University Press
McGraw-Hill Education
McGraw-Hill House
Shoppenhangers Road
Maidenhead
Berkshire
England
SL6 2QL

email: enquiries@openup.co.uk
world wide web: www.openup.co.uk

and Two Penn Plaza, New York, NY 10121—2289, USA

First published 2008

A catalogue record of this book is available from the British Library

ISBN-13: 978-0-335-22214-8 (pb) 978-0-335-22215-5 (hb)
ISBN-10: 0-335-22214-5 (pb) 0-335-22215-3 (hb)

Typeset by Kerrypress, Luton, Bedfordshire
Printed and bound in the UK by Bell and Bain Ltd, Glasgow

The McGraw·Hill Companies

CONTENTS

THE CONTRIBUTORS

Sarah Banks is a professor in the School of Applied Social Sciences at Durham University. She has written extensively on professional ethics, including *Ethics and Values in Social Work* (3rd edn, Palgrave Macmillan 2006) and *Ethics, Accountability and the Social Professions* (Palgrave Macmillan 2004). She qualified as a social worker in the mid-1980s and has worked in statutory and voluntary sector community development. She currently teaches on professional qualifying programmes in community and youth work and is working on research projects on professional integrity in social welfare and the role of faith communities in work with young people.

Peter Beresford took up his first post at Brunel University in 1990 as a senior lecturer in social policy. He became a professor in 1998 and currently holds a number of posts including Director of the Centre for Citizen Participation, Chair of Shaping our Lives, Visiting Fellow at the School for Social Work and Psycho-social studies at the University of East Anglia, and Fellow of the Royal Society of Arts. He is also a trustee of the Social Care Institute for Excellence. Professor Beresford is widely recognized for his contribution to the field. In particular, he has taken a leading role in developing new directions in user engagement in research at a time when there is growing political and research interest in this issue. He highlights the need to approach service user involvement in research critically and systematically, taking account of the diversity of approaches that have developed.

Lena Dominelli is Professor of Applied Social Sciences and an academician in the Academy of the Learned Societies for Social Sciences. She is an experienced educator, practitioner and researcher and has published extensively in the fields of sociology, social policy and social work. Among her most recent books are: *Broadening Horizons: International Exchanges in Social Work* (2003); *Social Work: Theory and Practice in a Changing Profession* (2004); *Social Work Futures: Transforming Theory and Practice in Social Work* (2005); and *Women and Community Action* (2006). She has received accolades for her contributions to social welfare in the international arena, including a medal from the Social Affairs Committee of the French Senate.

Michael Flood is a postdoctoral fellow at La Trobe University, Australia. He is also a trainer and community educator with a long involvement in community advocacy and education focused on men's violence against women. In 2006, he received a New South Wales Violence Against Women Prevention Award for his role in raising community and professional awareness of violence prevention.

Joan Healey is a senior lecturer in occupational therapy at Sheffield Hallam University. She has worked for many years with older people in health and social care settings and has undertaken research into service integration and service user empowerment in services for older people. She has a special interest in reflective and creative writing as an educational approach to enhancing practice-based learning. She is co-author of *Surviving your Placement in Health and Social Care: A Student Guide* (Open University Press 2008).

Ray Jones is a registered social worker. From 1992 to 2006 he was Director of Social Services, and then Director of Adult and Community Services in Wiltshire. He was the first chief executive of the Social Care Institute for Excellence and has been deputy chair, and then chair, of the British Association of Social Workers. He is a visiting professor at the University of Bath (and previously at the University of Exeter), an honorary fellow of the University of Gloucestershire. He is the author of five books, and numerous published papers, on social work and social policy.

Bill Jordan is Professor of Social Policy at Plymouth, Huddersfield and London Metropolitan Universities. He was a social worker for 20 years, an activist in a poor people's movement, and has held visiting chairs in Germany, the Netherlands, Denmark, Slovakia, Hungary and Australia. He is the author of 25 books on social policy, social work and politics.

Beth E. Richie is Professor of African American Studies and Criminology at the University of Illinois, Chicago. As a social worker and a sociologist, the focus of her work has been on responding to issues of racism, gender violence and other forms of social disadvantage. She is the author of numerous articles and the book, *Compelled to Crime: The Gender Entrapment of Black Battered Women.* Dr Richie is an activist committed to social justice as well as an academic committed to engaged scholarship on women, race and violence.

George Ritzer is Distinguished University Professor at the University of Maryland. His books include *The McDonaldization of*

Society (5th edn, 2008), *Enchanting a Disenchanted World* (2nd edn, 2005) and *The Globalization of Nothing* (2nd edn, 2007). He is currently working on *The Outsourcing of Everything* (with Craig Lair, forthcoming). His books have been translated into over 20 languages, with over a dozen translations of *The McDonaldization of Society*.

Vishanthie Sewpaul is a senior professor and head of the School of Social Work and Community Development, University of KwaZulu Natal (UKZN), Durban. She is chair of the Association of South African Social Work Educators' Institutions (ASASWEI); serves on the board of the International Associations of Schools of Social Work (IASSW), and is President of the National Association of Social Workers (South Africa). She was chair of the Global Standards Committee and has presented keynote addresses, papers and workshops at various local, national and international conferences, as well as publishing widely. She is regarded as one of the most prestigious researchers at UKZN, and is currently the deputy editor of *International Social Work*. She has special interests in the areas of globalization and social policy, emancipatory pedagogy and gender, AIDS and sexuality.

THE EDITORS

Dr Adam Barnard is a senior lecturer in Human Services in the Division of Social Work, Health and Social Care, and Counselling at Nottingham Trent University. He combines his academic interest in critical social theory with DIY cultural activism. He has been teaching, lecturing and researching for 15 years, and his research interests include critical social theory, moral philosophy and values, political philosophy with particular reference to post-war France, and existential and humanistic philosophy. He is currently engaged in a range of empirical research projects and theoretical reflection.

Nigel Horner is Deputy Head of Social Work at Lincoln University, where he teaches social work history, theory and methods, and children's services practice. He began working in a London borough children's home in 1972, before studying sociology at Durham University. After a period as a community worker, he qualified in social work from Glasgow University in 1980, and thereafter worked in mental health, child guidance, fostering and youth offending settings. He is the author of *What is Social Work?*

Jim Wild is a senior lecturer at Nottingham Trent University, convener of the Unit for Critical Studies in Men and Masculinities and course leader for the Diploma in Applied Studies in Working with Men. He is an activist and was instrumental in organizing the largest gatherings in social work and social care through successive conferences on the value base of social work and social care in 2006 and 2008 which were hosted by Nottingham Trent University's School of Social Work, Health and Social Care and Counselling. He also teaches on values and safeguarding children. His forthcoming publication 'Foundations for Good Practice in Safeguarding Children and Young People' will also be published with Open University Press later in 2008.

FOREWORD

by Camila Batmanghelidjh of Kids Company

On 2 March, 2006 I was invited to deliver a keynote paper in Nottingham relating to the conference, 'Affirming Our Value Base in Social Work and Social Care'. I had not been to Nottingham before. I am invited to speak at many conferences, but there is often a tendency for the organizers to make exaggerated claims about how their event will go, the number of people who will attend and so on. So when Jim Wild said almost 2000 people would turn up I was anxious that, not only had I accepted to speak at another event when I should be focused on my charity, Kids Company, but I was also going to a conference organized by someone who was unduly optimistic but also slightly deluded – 2000 people in our profession willing to go to a conference on values in the year 2006? Get real! However, when I arrived at the Royal Concert Hall I discovered that he was right – well, there were 1982 individuals in the hall so I still think he was exaggerating! It was truly wonderful to see all those faces in front of me – students, practitioners and academics all together. The event made me think about values, the sort of society we want, the sort of society *we need*. Daily in the newspapers we hear reports about a pending environmental catastrophe and I cannot help but find parallels between the work I do with young people on the edge of their identity – abused, neglected and reviled, reaching out for help in ways that often result in rejection and hostility – and the denial mechanisms we use to shelter ourselves from an ecological breakdown. There seem to be psychological mechanisms that 'kick in' when we face danger and hostility, or when our comfort zone is challenged.

After the event in Nottingham I felt more than ever that an understanding of a value base in social care is needed to deliver quality and reduce confusion and despair. It is something to which I have given a great deal of thought. There are several ways to approach a definition of our value base in the care professions and one could begin with a list of desired characteristics. It is likely to be a long list, commencing with a right to dignity, and moving on to embrace issues of justice, anti-discrimination, honesty, integrity, reliability and the championing of equalities. But these concepts become diluted when seen through the lens of our modernization agenda, with its focus on professionalism, accountability, cost codes, units, statistical data, budget under-spends, overspends, time management, appraisal, continual pro-fessional development ... and before you know it we have the corruption of our desire to care and make a difference. Often our managers and commissioners are so removed from front-line realities that to combat individualism, community disintegration and indifference we have to 'teach' what it's like to be good and effective workers. How impoverished a society is that?

The trouble with 'modernized' structures is that practitioners can find themselves overwhelmed and disillusioned very quickly. It is like a recipe book that is too thick and impossible to fathom – full of 'statutory' guidelines mixed with free market notions of caring, and with an eye on a balance sheet. So as the service user screams obscenities down the phone, hits their fist on the reception desk, or looks you straight in the eye and lies, how do you access your value base? Some service users who have been neglected and traumatized harbour greater challenges. They may be struggling with multiple oppressions, sometimes have unproc-essed traumatic memories and experience ongoing discrimination, which often leads them to seek resolution through impulsive acts of revenge or violence.

The difficulty with current trends across health and social care services is that administrative functions have become the primary focus because, as outcomes and outputs, they are *easier* to measure than human distress. Managers can feel secure counting the visits, signing off forms, ticking boxes and documenting meetings. Yet, despite ever increasing efficiencies, social care is losing out to its own outrageous obsessions with accountability and control. The aspirational young worker soon learns to assume neutrality, which enables a safe disguise; a kind of facelessness emerges, ensuring that in the 'watch your back' under-resourced, blame-led culture you do not become the target. A discrepancy develops between the fire in the belly – that emotional desire to care (which in the first place drove the worker into the profes-sion) – and the reality of daily work which is delivered in a sanitized context of personal survival.

The service user can be confused by the mechanized emo-tional coldness of the worker and the worker can be immobilized and dejected by an inability to live out something meaningful within the workplace. Both are looking for something significant in the contact and both are denied it. In the process, an insidious emotional death blankets the contact.

So might I dare to suggest that old fashioned words like 'love', 'compassion' and 'empathy' need to be unleashed with potential through all our lives? Every time you meet a service user, try to honour the essence of your value base; then there is no need to be vigilant about a long list of commandments and warnings. In an increasingly globalized world, where human endeavour has a price and market forces corrupt our notion of human existence, hold on to fundamental principles and notions of what makes us become effective in our work, and resist that terrible controlling model of 'care' which seems to subvert the very essence of what we need to be great workers who truly make a difference. I commend this publication, which attempts to make a stand against those forces because, in the end, if we have no values in society, what do we have?

Leaving you with a recommendation to love.

Camila Batmanghelidjh, founder, Kids Company

INTRODUCTION

People everywhere – under very different conditions – are asking themselves where are we? What are we living through? Where are we being taken? What have we lost? How do we continue without a plausible vision of the future? Why have we lost any view of what is beyond a life-time?

Berger (2007: 36)

Not everyone necessarily thinks like John Berger, but the above quote from his wonderful book could actually relate quite well to social work and the social care professions, as well as to existential reflections on a world increasingly defined without meaning, sustenance or identity.

Social care employers seem less concerned with values and ethics – which we can argue, should form the foundations of what are central attributes to our work – and more with assuring that the workforce possesses the appropriate attributes, competences and skills necessary to be able to perform tasks in accordance with defined occupational standards and nationally prescribed performance indicators.

Within this atmosphere of organizational and service uniformity, Lymbery and Postle (2007: 3) suggest that 'practitioners must therefore retain clarity about their role and contribution to welfare services and be prepared to argue for the continuing relevance of their role within work environments that they may find harsh and unforgiving'.

As a response to this challenge, it has long been felt that it is social work's distinctive *value base* that best exemplifies and advances the profession's identity and historic purpose, and hence the intrinsic rationale of this important text. Indeed, we should acknowledge that it has been social work which has pioneered many of the debates and ideas which are now commonplace in wider areas of social care.

In one sense, it has been recognized that social work is a chameleon–like activity, with the apparent capacity to change its identity to suit its purchaser. It appears to be easily bought, readily switching from an emancipatory, liberationist position to one of social control and regulation. As Howe (2002: 86) observes, 'In the broadest sense, the purposes of social work are determined by prevailing political ideologies'; and the Quality Assurance Agency (QAA) *Social Work Benchmark Statement* (2000: 2.2.3) affirms that 'Social work adapts and changes in response to social, political and economic challenges and the demands of contemporary social welfare policy, practice and legislation'.

So are we engaged in a fruitless search for certainty and consistency, where there is none? Are we constantly changing themes, ideas and beliefs?

As a small contribution to the debate on the 5th of March 2006 and 1st of March 2008, Nottingham Trent University, in conjunction with our Regional Social Work Network and national organisations including BASW, SWAP and Community Care, embarked on plans to organize an activist-based events on the value base of social work and social care. Values have taken a dip in popularity over the past 20 years; they have been eroded, deferred to backwater debates and are no longer seen as part of a wider 'competence'-based agenda. We wondered – would people come? That first event in 2006 proved to be one of the largest in social work and social care conferences in recent history, with almost 2000 individuals attending. As he stood on the stage in awe at the sea of faces before him, Bob Holman, who chaired the first morning, enthusiastically claimed, 'It's like being back in the 1970s!'

Indeed, the event was not so much a reflection back, but more an acknowledgement that at such a time where values are so fractured and disregarded in our work *there is* possibly a resurgence and enthusiasm for such fundamental issues in our profession.

The keynote speakers who contributed their valuable and creative thoughts, beliefs and observations to the conferences and subsequent collection of chapters are all wedded to a particular belief in the capacity of social work and social care to liberate itself from the dead hand of bureaucratic control, and to reaffirm its commitment to a value base that seeks to address the needs of individual members of society, while equally addressing and challenging the structural processes that either created or exacerbated those very individual needs. Their perspectives are varied, their focus diverse and their solutions not necessarily consistent. But they agree that social work has a distinctive contribution to make, and that it needs to advance its potential through a wider range of activities.

We hope the range and scope of the chapters that follow will help students and practitioners acknowledge that values contribute to all activities in social work and social care; that activities of multinational companies are as concerning as the experiences of the service user who seeks an inclusive service based on collaboration and respect.

We also hope that the exercises at the end of each chapter will be used to assist teaching and learning in a creative and 'active' approach to defining values.

The following chapters do not offer any easy answers – because there aren't any. They will serve, hopefully, to reinvigorate social work's identity and its commitment to a set of values that will serve its service users perhaps more than itself.

References

Berger, J. (2007) *Hold Everything Dear: Dispatches on Survival and Resistance.* London: Verso.

Howe, D. (2002) Relating theory to practice, in M. Davies (ed.) *The Blackwell Companion to Social Work*, 2nd edn. Oxford: Blackwell.

Lymbery, M. and Postle, K. (2007) Social work: a companion for learning – an introduction, in M. Lymbery and K. Postle (eds) *Social Work: A Companion to Learning.* London: Sage.

QAA (Quality Assurance Agency) (2000) *Social Work Benchmark Statement.* Gloucester: Quality Assurance Agency for Higher Education.

chapter **one**

VALUES, ETHICS AND PROFESSIONALIZATION: A SOCIAL WORK HISTORY

Adam Barnard

It has long been argued that social work is a value-based and professional activity. In the field of professional ethics, 'values' usually take the form of general ethical principles relating to how professionals should treat the people they work with and what sorts of actions are regarded as right or wrong. Vigilante (1974) calls values the 'fulcrum of practice'; Bernstein (1970) suggests that they offer 'vision and discernment'; and Younghusband (1967) suggests they are 'everywhere in practice'. Timms (1983) pleaded for 'value-talk' to be central in social work. Values have a rich and detailed history and an exploration of the historical emergence of those values allows us to gain some purchase on the present, and to explore contemporary controversies and dilemmas.

There are four spheres of values within social work. The first is the more abstract field of moral philosophy that forms a backdrop to ethical debates in social work. The second is the distinct forms of legislation that have created the context for social work practice alongside providing legal responses to particular social work issues and cases. The third is the domain of political ideologies and the way that these have shaped and sculpted social work models, methods and practices. The final sphere is the historical emergence of social work as a profession and the struggle for a professional identity that has engaged social workers. Shardlow (2002: 32) refers to these spheres as extended (social work as a social activity), mid-range (nature of social work as a professional activity) and restricted (professional ethics and behaviour with clients) definitions of ethics and values. This chapter attempts to address the last sphere of values and provide a flavour of the debates that surround the developments in social work ethics. Broad reviews of ethics and moral philosophy can be found within Russell (1961), Hamlyn (1987), Rachels (2003) and Grayling (2004). Legislation is ably discussed by Brayne and Carrr (2003), while political ideologies are considered by Heywood (2005).

Firstly, a word on how we can understand the change in ideas about values. Thomas Kuhn's *The Structure of Scientific Revolutions* (1970) became one of the most influential books of the twentieth century. Kuhn, as a physicist turned philosopher of science, conducted research to teach a course on the history of science to humanities students at Harvard in the 1960s (Holloway 2005: 63). Kuhn's picture of the development of scientific ideas and, by extension, ideas in general, did not fit with the 'common sense' or 'customary' view. This would suggest that ideas develop in a piecemeal, evolutionary and cumulative way, each idea building on the contribution of previous generations. The £2 coin enshrines this view with a quotation, attributed to Isaac Newton, stamped on its rim. It reads: 'Standing on the shoulders of giants', suggesting that Newton's progress in ideas and intellectual development built on the previous achievements of great thinkers. Kuhn's work revolutionized this common-sense or customary view by suggesting that ideas develop in a much more dramatic and interruptive way. He used the term 'paradigm' to express the 'constellation of beliefs, assumptions and techniques' that hold sway at a given point in time. People are socialized into a paradigm and it becomes the accepted 'world view' or 'received idea' (Rojeck *et al.* 1988: 6) of a particular community. Paradigms dominate a period of 'normal science' where a community engages in simple puzzle-solving rather than raising any challenging or difficult questions about the paradigm itself. There is a high degree of social control in the adherence to the paradigm. The growth of anomalies, which do not fit this paradigm or received idea, stand out due to the strong attachment to a paradigm. Kuhn argues that when these anomalies become unbearable, science enters a period of crisis when a more far-reaching and speculative acceptance of a new paradigm emerges. This process results in a 'paradigm shift' or scientific revolution that overthrows the previous world of knowledge and replaces it with a new world view.

The classic paradigm shift in science was the move from Aristotelian to Copernican astronomy. The classical world view saw the cosmos as a series of concentric circles with the earth fixed at the centre. The planets moved around the earth with nothing beyond them except the realm of God (Holloway 2005: 65). This was the big story throughout Europe for centuries until the anomalies identified by Copernicus prompted the search for a new paradigm that could accommodate them. The Copernican revolution shifted the paradigm of the universe to locate the sun at the centre of our system and develop a 'helio-centric' world view. We could suggest Einstein overturned the world of Newton and brought about a new paradigm in physics. It is now widely accepted that a vision of a 'flat earth' is discredited and we accept the shifting ground of plate tectonics as the composition of the world.

Social work and its connection to the history of values

A further example of the power of the paradigm can be drawn from childcare policy. Lorraine Fox Harding (1997) has identified four paradigms or value positions in childcare policy. The first is the *laissez faire* and patriarchal approach applied up to the mid-nineteenth century that sought to preserve family privacy, and by which parents, particularly fathers, had power over children with minimal state intervention. The image of a disciplinarian Victorian patriarch held sway. This is 'the view that power in the family should not be disturbed except in extreme circumstances, and the role of the state should be a minimal one' (Fox Harding 1997: 9). Towards the end of the nineteenth century, state paternalism and child protection emerged. This saw the protection of children by an emerging group of (female) professionals, and is associated with the growth of state intervention as the twentieth century progressed. State intervention is often authoritarian, with the result that biological family bonds can be undervalued and good quality care substituted. Criticism of state paternalism in the post-Second World War period attempted to defend families from heavy-handed state intervention and offer greater levels of help and support. This saw 'kinship defenders or defence of the birth family' emerge as a dominant paradigm. The final paradigm in relation to child protection is the children's rights and child liberation perspective, in which children are seen as the bearers of rights and able to participate in decision-making processes.

Fox Harding's work shows the historic paradigmatic shifts of value positions in relation to childcare policy in social work theory and practice. Having examined the way in which ideas develop, we can turn our attention to the paradigm shifts that are evident in social work and social care values. We have provided a flavour of this process with Fox Harding, above, but will extend this argument. The following discussion examines the broad historical changes in values within social work, social care and human services. Further reading is provided at the end of the chapter for those wanting to examine the philosophical basis of values, ethics and social work.

There is a multitude of varied value systems that could have been selected. For example, the Arab world, Africa and China, have all contributed philosophical discussion to questions of values. However, in terms on the impact and contribution made to social work, the selection for discussion is always going to be partial. This is not to do a disservice to the contribution made by a diverse range of thinkers or to devalue the knowledge they have produced, but to map out a digestible survey of the terrain of values that have a continuing legacy in the helping and social professions. Useful and wider ranging commentaries on this subject are Yelaja (1970), Midgley (1981) and Osei-Hwedie (1990, 1993).

Social work values defined: an emerging story

The profession's early concern with the value of charity has its roots in the Bible and religion. All the world's religions uphold ethics of duty, mutual responsibility, care, compassion and concern for others (Horner 2006: 16). Reamer (2006: 15) argues that acts of charity were meant to fulfil God's commandments. The Elizabethan Poor Laws of 1598 and 1601 consolidated welfare legislation of the Tudor period and have their origins in the systems of relief provided to the poor by the parishes of the Church of England.

The seventeenth century saw the emergence of what we could call 'modern values', with the intellectual, cultural and political movement that is collectively referred to as the Enlightenment. This was characterized by an increased emphasis on the values of tolerance, freedom and reasonableness. Authoritarianism, particularly of a religious kind, was rejected in favour of respect for lay opinion, increased scepticism and a belief in progress, emancipation and scientific understanding (Brown 2003: 4). For some, social work stems from these roots (Payne 2005: 15).

Modern values have been concerned with addressing the questions, 'What is the right thing to do?' or 'How should I act?' Early contributors to such questions were Jeremy Bentham and John Stuart Mill. They developed an ethical system based on the consequences of action and hedonism, and the promotion of happiness as the basis of ethics. People should always act in ways that make the largest number of people happy. This form of utilitarianism (Bentham [1789] 1970; Mill [1848] 1972) had a significant impact on social, political and legal reform (Sen and Williams 1982; Glover 1990; Crisp 1997). Philosophically, the 1800s were significant in terms of Immanuel Kant's contribution. Kant's challenging philosophical system gives us an ethics based on duty, moral motivation and ultimately a respect for other people (Paton 1948).

During the Georgian period, social welfare systems were most concerned with the threat to public order presented by those in poverty. The workhouse was the eighteenth-century response, with 2000 existing in Britain by 1776 as a result of the General Workhouses Act of the 1720s (Horner 2006: 18). *The Poor Law Report* leading to the Poor Law Amendment Act in 1834 saw the consolidation of workhouses across the country, acting as harsh and deterring institutions encouraging moral restraint. Foucault (1961) refers to this as the 'great confinement' that spread across Europe from the mid-seventeenth century and found its fullest expression in the 'institutional mania' of the Victorian era (Horner 2006: 19). 'Lunatics, idiots and imbeciles' were confined to institutions, away from the celebratory grandeur of Victorian public buildings. Horner (2006: 21) suggests that this period threw up a range of middle-class reformers including Elizabeth Fry, Florence Nightingale, Mary Carpenter, Octavia Hill, Dr Barnardo, General Booth, Edwin Chadwick, Edward Foster, Dr Thomas Arnold and Lord Shaftesbury. Although moral education was part of these reformers' programmes there was a growing awareness of other sources of difficulty for people. By 1900, the essentially religious base to charity gave way to secular ideas of social welfare.

Reamer (2006) provides an insight into the historical emergence of the values base in social care. Values and ethics have been the cornerstone of social care's mission and have involved normative considerations of what should be done in terms of its ethical orientation. Reamer argues that the evolution of social work values and ethics has had four distinct stages: the morality period; the values period; the ethical theory and decision-making period; and the ethical standards and risk management period (2006: 5).

The morality period, when social work became a profession, was more concerned with the morality of the client than with the values of the practitioner. Responding to the 'curse of pauperism' (Paine 1880) and organizing relief was the principle mission. Reamer (2006: 5) suggests that this led to paternalistic attempts to strengthen the moral rectitude of 'wayward' clients, and social reforms reflected this – for example, the 'settlement house' movements in the USA. The Society for Organizing Charitable Relief and Repressing Mendicity, later to become the Charity Organization Societies in the UK, aimed to raise the moral stature of individuals and society (Bisman 2003). 'The most important insight charity organizers left us was their view of society as a moral community ... a body of people held together primarily by intimate sentiments of responsibility, love and duty, caring and sharing' (Leiby 1984: 535). These moral concerns laid the foundations for some of the primary values of social work, emphasizing the importance of individual worth and dignity, and service to humanity (Bisman 2003: 112).

The early part of the twentieth century saw a shift in concern from the morality of the client towards the structural problems of society such as housing, healthcare, sanitation, employment and poverty. In a UK context this culminated in the *Beveridge Report* of 1942 that declared a 'War on Want' to address these structural problems. An emerging class of welfare professionals developed what we might call 'traditional social work'.

'Traditional' social work is seen as 'the technical management of personal problems and the maintenance of order' (Rojeck *et al.* 1988: 1) and has normally been composed of 'received ideas' relating to professional values and standards of practice. These have often taken a list-type approach. Biesteck, a Catholic priest, drew up one of the early and influential list-type approaches to practice that included: individualization; the purposeful expression of feelings; controlled emotional involvement; acceptance; non-judgemental attitude; client self-determination; and confidentiality (Biesteck 1957).

In the USA in the 1950s, the National Association of Social Workers (NASW 1958) listed social work's basic values as: respect for 'individual uniqueness'; the right to 'the realization of the full potential of each individual'; and tolerance of 'the differences that exist between individuals' (Rojeck *et al.* 1988: 6). The main opposition to this approach developed in the 1960s with radical social work, a broad church that drew from labelling theory, critical psychoanalysis, Marxism, feminism and discourse theory. The criticism of traditional social work was that it held an ahistorical view of social work values and neglected the context in which social values emerge and change. A further criticism was that the structural forces which give rise to personal and social problems were being neglected (Rojeck *et al.* 1988: 2).

The radical challenge emerges

Humanism and existentialism also exerted an influence as well as being established philosophical theories. Humanism argues that human beings have the capacity to reason, make choices and act freely, independent of religion. Payne (2005: 182) argues that humanism gained favour as part of the secularization of welfare that separated it from the churches in the 1800s. Carl Rogers (1951, 1961) is the most influential writer on humanistic and person-centred ideas. He suggests three elements to relationships, stating that clients should perceive workers as genuine and congruent (reflecting real attitudes and a personality not imposed on clients), that workers should have unconditional positive regard for clients, and that they should have empathy for clients.

Existentialism is built on the notion of humans as free, unique individuals whose 'existence precedes essence'. Sartre's imperious *Being and Nothingness* (1943) is focused on this notion of free will and the meaning that people create. Existentialism's contribution to social work came through the anti-psychiatry movement and the work of R.D. Laing. Its fullest recent application to social work is by Thompson (1992).

By the 1960s social work as a profession had become self-reflective and the 'values clarification' movement (Reamer 2006: 6) examined the value base of social work. It drew on developments in related disciplines such as psychotherapy and social policy, and from social and political struggles such as the civil rights movements and women's liberation. Social workers became more reflective about their own value base and their relationship to the profession. Social work training examined a broad set of emancipatory issues such as social equality, welfare rights, discrimination and oppression.

In a UK context, radical social work informed by Marxist social and political theory viewed received ideas of 'care' and 'concern' as part of social work's historical mission to aid capitalism by ensuring a compliant and healthy workforce and addressing the worst excesses of capitalism (Corrigan and Leonard 1978). The ideological smokescreen of social work was to 'blame the victim' and locate social problems as instances of individual failing, not structurally defined problems. The central concern of the value base of radical social work was a focus on equality, understood in the Marxist sense of redistribution of income and wealth, and a notion of justice built on that redistribution. Bailey and Brake (1975, 1980) argue that radical practice is 'essentially understanding the position of the oppressed in the context of the social and economic structure they live in' (Bailey and Brake 1975: 9). Marxist-informed social work was criticized by feminists for focusing too heavily on class and for neglecting the family, gender, sexuality, patriarchy and domestic violence, as well as questions of culture and ethnicity (Ahmed 1990; Martin and Martin 1995).

The 1970s saw a surge of interest in the broad subject of applied or professional ethics, that Reamer (2006: 6) suggests also influenced social work ethics. High profile cases of social work failure consolidated this process. The 'ethical theory and decision-making' period characterized this boom in applied ethics and greater ethical consideration. In terms of social work ethics, Plant's *Social and Moral Theory in Casework* (1970) represents one of the first sustained attempts to examine the philosophical value base of social work. Previous attempts had been less philosophically informed (Biestek 1957; Hollis 1964) and took the form of 'list approaches' to the types of values to which social workers should be committed. Hunt (1978) attempted a philosophically justified examination of the value base of social work and suggests that it is comprised of the uniqueness and worth of each individual human personality, the right to self-determination, the existence and value of freedom, the existence of obligations, plus a host of beliefs about the 'good life' and 'good society'.

In 1970s Britain, the British Association of Social Workers (BASW 1975) drew up a list in their code of ethics that included the principles of 'self-determination', 'non-judgementalism', 'compassion', 'professional responsibility' and 'confidentiality'. The end of this era was signalled, for Payne (2005: 233), by the general political developments in many western countries that gave rise to the 'New Right' of Conservative administrations. Conservative approaches to social values are built on the two tenets that the individual is paramount and that private activity should address social problems. Individual failures are to blame for a person's situation although there is a key role for the family and society's morality in socializing individuals into the correct forms of behaviour.

The 1980s was 'a watershed moment that dramatically changed social workers' understanding of and approach to ethical issues' (Reamer 2006: 9). The Barclay Report (1982: 145) into the future of social work argued that social workers should work in ways that recognize people have a need for 'respect', 'understanding', 'justice' and 'equality'. Respect (the value of the innate dignity and worth of human persons), individualization (the uniqueness of individuals), and confidentiality were central to the language of social work (Timms 1983; Clark and Asquith 1985). From the 1980s onwards there was a growing concern for social work to respond to ethnic and cultural dimensions by addressing anti-oppressive approaches and cultural and ethnic sensitivity (Thompson 1993, 2003a, 2003b; Darymple and Burke 1995; Dominelli 1997, 2002).

Developments in philosophy and social theory have also contributed to the paradigmatic change in social work values. Discourse analysis has displaced the idea that the language of social work is neutral or a formal and technical exercise of intervention into people's lives. The notion of discourse suggests that power relations are inherent in language and help to shape the reality that individuals and groups inhabit. As such, language is central to the power of social work – for example, by defining people as 'abnormal', 'deviant', 'delinquent' or 'at risk'. The simplest example of this is to consider the terms 'man' and 'woman'. Woman is comprised of 'man' 'wo(man)', she always needs 'man' to be present to define herself, man comes first. French poststructuralist philosophers who have informed discourse theory, such as Jacques Derrida (1976), suggest that to clearly display the power relations inherent in social life, 'man' should be written as 'wo(man)'. Women are presented as passive, maternal, submissive, docile, virtuous and emotional whereas men are active, businesslike, decisive, rational and reasonable (Spender 1980). Postmodernism, 'not so much a theoretical perspective as a style of theorizing' (Thompson 2003b: 55) is the culmination of these developments.

The contemporary situation in the helping professions

The 1990s saw the emergence of a further paradigmatic approach with anti-oppression, empowerment and advocacy emerging as themes. Anti-oppressive practice (Thompson 1993; Dominelli 1996) locates the worker and service user in a broader structural context, focusing on social difference, personal and political relationships, power, history and reflexivity (Clifford 1995). Empowerment involves supporting service users to identify the full range of possibilities, strengths and qualities required to meet their needs. Solomon (1976), Lee (2001) and Gutiérrez *et al.* (1998) are representative of attempts to develop empowerment as a central approach as well as a fundamental value. Advocacy as a positive sense of self, knowledge, and strategies to gain goals is central to Rose and Black's (1985) argument, and Brandon *et al.* (1995) placed this value at the heart of modern social work and social care.

Professional competences have also added to the present climate of social work values such as compassion, discernment, trustworthiness, integrity and conscientiousness. Compassion is a trait that combines an active regard for another's welfare with an awareness and emotional response of sympathy, tenderness and discomfort at another's misfortune (Reamer 2006: 31). Discernment is being able to bring 'sensitive insight, acute judgement, and understanding into action' without prejudice (Reamer 2006: 31). Trustworthiness is the reliance on another person to act with the right motives and appropriate moral norms (Reamer 2006: 31). Integrity refers to the soundness, wholeness and reliability of the moral character of an individual who has a coherent understanding of themselves in terms of their emotions, aspirations and knowledge, with a commitment to moral norms (Reamer 2006: 31). Being conscientious is to do what is right and exerting appropriate effort to do so (Reamer 2006: 32). These are focal virtues that Beauchamp and Childress (2001) offer as critically important in work carried out by professionals.

There are dangers in this type of list approach in that it leaves practitioners with little more than a set of fixed values that they should bring into complex situations. Beauchamp and Childress (2001) argue that such values are linked to four core moral principles. *Autonomy* is self-direction and self-rule free from controlling interference. It is to become an author of your own destiny free from the control of others. *Nonmaleficence* is the obligation to do no harm to others. *Beneficence* includes altruism, love and humanity and connotes acts of kindness, mercy and charity (Reamer 2006: 32). *Justice* is a difficult term that refers to fairness, equity and appropriate treatment in the light of what is owed to a person. It is closely connected to equality and rights. This cluster of values includes professional competencies and core moral principles that cover Shardlow's (2002) expansive, mid-range and restrictive values.

The most recent stage of social work ethics is the maturation of ethical issues and the significant expansion of ethical standards to guide a practitioner's conduct and increased knowledge concerning professional negligence and liability (Reamer 2006: 9). The risk management period has been consolidated by events such as the General Social Care Council's code of conduct for social care workers. This code (General Social Care Council 2004) contains six statements that should guide and inform social work's values and social workers' practice. These are:

1 Protect the rights and promote the interests of service users and carers.
2 Strive to establish and maintain the trust and confidence of service users and carers.

3   Promote the independence of service users while protecting them as far as possible from danger or harm.
4   Respect the rights of service users while seeking to ensure that their behaviour does not harm themselves or other people.
5   Uphold public trust and confidence in social care services.
6   Be accountable for the quality of your work and take responsibility for maintaining and improving your knowledge and skills.

The changing nature of social care, human services and social professions has promoted two further contemporary developments in values. The first is the trend towards 'interprofessional' working. Collaborative working arrangements mean that problems or services are addressed or delivered by groups of professionals working together. Health visitors, social workers, educational psychologists, and the police would be one example of interprofessional working. Regeneration partnerships to tackle social problems within a community or neighbourhood often involve 'interagency' working between professionals. The 'modernization' or 'modern management agenda' of New Labour places a stress on 'joined up' policy and practice. This interprofessional working demands a focus on the values of each profession and the possibility of conflicting values between each profession.

Similarly, more defensive ways of working have emerged. Banks (2004: 8) argues that the 'new accountability' encapsulates a host of accountability measures that have developed with the growth of 'new managerialism' or 'new public management' from the end of the twentieth century. Major changes in the delivery of welfare and the introduction of internal markets pose interesting challenges for the values base of professions working in social care. Working with first-year students there is a worrying trend towards what Reamer (2006: 19) calls an 'amoralistic paradigm'. This is characterized by the absence of value-based or normative concepts or orientations and is evident in a technical, managerial or procedural approach to social work. The act of 'rule-following' or upholding a duty to the regulatory framework, uncritically and without question, would be an example of such amoralistic working. The concern is that contemporary developments in the field of social care have returned us to the starting point of traditional social work as the technical management of personal problems and the maintenance of order. The challenge is to move beyond this paradigm and reinvigorate the value base of social care. The challenges of globalization, new technologies, regulation and government policy will set the agenda for new developments in how we define values.

To return to the notion of a paradigm shift in professional values, Banks (2004) argues that changes in values have 'not signalled a revolution' but a 'series of tremors, rocking the foundations, requiring some rebuilding and restructuring, but based on the solid traditions of the past, constantly evolving and changing' (p. 194). It is this common but shifting ground that makes up the terrain of values. Our task is to map the route and enjoy the journey.

References

Ahmed, B. (1990) *Black Perspectives in Social Work*. Birmingham: Venture.

Bailey, R. and Brake, M. (eds) (1975) *Radical Social Work*. London: Edward Arnold.

Bailey, R. and Brake, M. (eds) (1980) *Radical Social Work and Practice*. London: Edward Arnold.

Banks, S. (2004) *Ethics, Accountability and the Social Professions*. London: Palgrave.

Barclay Report (1982) *Social Workers, their Roles and Tasks*. London: Bedford Square Press.

BASW (British Association of Social Workers) (1975) A code of ethics for social work, in D. Watson (ed.) *A Code of Ethics for Social Work: The Second Step*. London: RKP.

Beauchamp, T. and Childress, J. (2001) *Principles of Biomedical Ethics*, 5th edn. New York: Oxford University Press.

Bentham, J. ([1789] 1970) *An Introduction to the Principles of Morals and Legislation*. London: Athelone Press.

Bernstein, S. (1970) *Further Explorations in Groupwork*. London: Bookstall.

Biesteck, F. (1957) *The Casework Relationship*. London: George Allen & Unwin.

Bisman, C. (2003) Social work values: the moral core of the profession, *British Journal of Social Work*, 34(1): 9–123.

Brandon, D., Brandon, A. and Brandon, T. (1995) *Advocacy: Power to People with Disabilities*. Birmingham: Venture.

Brayne, H. and Carr, H. (2003) *Law for Social Workers*, 8th edn. Oxford: Oxford University Press

Brown, S. (ed.) (2003) *British Philosophy and the Age of Enlightenment*. London: Routledge.

Clark, C. and Asquith, S. (1985) *Social Work and Social Philosophy*. London: RKP.

Clifford, D.J. (1995) Methods in oral history and social work, *Journal of the Oral History Society*, 23(2).

Corrigan, P. and Leonard, P. (1978) *Social Work Practice under Capitalism: A Marxist Approach.* London: Palgrave Macmillan.

Crisp, R. (1997) *Mill on Utilitarianism.* London: Routledge.

Dalrymple, J. and Burke, B. (1995) *Anti-oppressive Practice: Social care and the Law.* Buckingham: Open University Press.

Derrida, J. (1976) *Of Grammatology.* Baltimore, MA: John Hopkins University Press.

Dominelli, L. (1996) Deprofessionalising social work: anti-oppressive practice, competencies and post-modernism, *British Journal of Social Work*, 26: 153–75.

Dominelli, L. (1997) *Anti-Racist Social Work Theory*, 2nd edn. Basingstoke: Palgrave.

Dominelli, L. (2002) *Anti-Oppressive Social Work Theory and Practice.* Basingstoke: Palgrave.

Foucault, M. (1961) *Folie de deraison: histoire de la folie à l'age classique.* Paris: Plon.

Fox Harding, L. (1997) *Perspectives in Child Care Policy*, 2nd edn. London: Longman.

General Social Care Council (2004) *Codes of Practice.* London: General Social Care Council.

Glover, J. (ed.) (1990) *Utilitarianism and its Critics.* London: Macmillan.

Grayling, A.C. (2004) *What is Good? The Search for the Best way to Live.* London: Phoenix.

Gutiérrez, L.M., Parsons, R.J. and Cox, E.O. (1998) *Empowerment in Social Work Practice: A Source Book.* Pacific Grove, CA: Brooks/Cole.

Hamlyn, D.W. (1987) *The Penguin History of Western Philosophy.* Harmondsworth: Penguin.

Heywood, A. (2005) *Political Ideologies.* London: Palgrave.

Hollis, F. (1964) *Casework: A Psychosocial Therapy.* New York: Random House.

Holloway, R. (2005) *Looking in the Distance: The Human Search for Meaning.* Edinburgh: Canongate.

Horner, N. (2006) *What is Social Work: Context and Perspectives*, 2nd edn. Exeter: Learning Matters.

Hunt, L. (1978) Social work and ideology, in N. Timms and D. Watson (eds) *Philosophy in Social Work.* London: RKP.

Kuhn, T. (1970) *The Structure of Scientific Revolutions.* Chicago: Chicago University Press.

Lee, J.A.B. (2001) *The Empowerment Approach to Social Work: Building the Beloved Community.* New York: Columbia University Press.

Leiby, J. (1984) Charity organization reconsidered, *Social Service Review*, December: 52–38.

Martin, E.P. and Martin, J.M. (1995) *Social Work and the Black Experience.* Washington: NASW Press.

Midgley (1981) *Professional Imperialism: Social Work in the Third World.* London: Heinemann.

Mill, J.S. ([1848] 1972) *Utilitarianism, Liberty, Representative Government.* London: Dent.

NASW (National Association of Social Workers) (1958) Working definitions of social work practice, *Social Work*, 3(April): 5–9.

Osei-Hwedie, K. (1990) Social work and the question of social development in Africa, *Journal of Social Development in Africa*, 5(2): 87–99.

Osei-Hwedie, K. (1993) The challenge of social work in Africa: starting the indigenization process, *Journal of Social Development in Africa*, 8(1): 19–30.

Paine, R.T. Jr. (1880) The work of volunteer visitors of the Associated Charities among the poor, *Journal of Social Science*, 12: 113.

Paton, H.J. (trans.) (1948) *The Moral Law: Kant's Groundwork on the Metaphysics of Morals*. London: Hutchinson.

Payne, M. (2005) *Modern Social Work Theory*, 3rd edn. London: Palgrave.

Plant, R. (1970) *Social and Moral Theory in Casework*. London: RKP.

Rachels, J. (2003) *The Elements of Philosophy*. London: McGraw-Hill.

Reamer, F.G. (2006) *Social Work Values and Ethics*, 2nd edn. New York: Columbia University Press.

Rogers, C. (1951) *Client-centred Therapy: Its Current Practice, Implications and Theory*. London: Constable.

Rogers, C. (1961) *On Becoming a Peron: A Therapist's View of Psychotherapy*. London: Constable.

Rojeck, C., Peacock, G. and Collins, S. (1988) *Social Work and Received Ideas*. London: Routledge.

Rose, S.M. and Black, B.L. (1985) *Advocacy and Empowerment: Mental Health Care in the Community*. Boston, MA: Routledge & Kegan Paul.

Russell, B. (1961) *History of Western Philosophy*. London: George Allen & Unwin.

Sartre, J.P. (1943) *Being and Nothingness*, trans. H. Barnes. London: Methuen.

Sen, A. and Williams, B.A.O. (eds) (1982) *Utilitarianism and Beyond*. Cambridge: Cambridge University Press.

Shardlow, S. (2002) Values, ethics and social work, in R. Adams, L. Dominelli and M. Payne (eds) (2002) *Social Work: Themes, Issues and Critical Debates*, 2nd edn. London: Palgrave.

Solomon, J. (1976) *Black Empowerment: Social Work in Oppressed Communities*. New York: Columbia University Press.

Spender, D. (1980) *Man Made Language*. London: RKP.

Thompson, N. (1992) *Existentialism and Social Work*. Aldershot: Avebury.

Thompson, N. (1993) *Anti-Discriminatory Practice*. London: Macmillan.

Thompson, N. (2003a) *Anti-Discriminatory Practice*, 3rd edn. Basingstoke: Palgrave.

Thompson, N. (2003b) *Promoting Equality: Challenging Discrimination and Oppression in the Human Services*. Basingstoke: Macmillan.

Timms, N. (1983) *Social Work Values: An Enquiry*. London: Routledge & Kegan Paul.

Vigilante, J. (1974) Between values and science: education for the professional during a moral crisis or is proof truth? *Journal of Education for Social Work*, 10(3): 107–15.

Yelaja, S.A. (1970) Towards a conceptualization of the social work profession in India, *Applied Social Studies*, 2(1): 21–6.

Younghusband, E. (1967) *Social Work and Social Values*. London: Allen & Unwin.

Further reading

Those wishing to pursue the philosophical basis to the emergence of values can consult Bertrand Russell's imperious *History of Western Philosophy* (1961, London: George Allen & Unwin) or Hamlyn's (1987) accessible *The Penguin History of Western Philosophy*. Lighter introductions to systems of philosophical thought, although without an explicit focus on values, are Gaarder, J. (1995) *Sophie's World: A Novel About the History of Philosophy* (London: Pheonix) and Pirsig, R. (1974) *Zen and the Art of Motor Cycle Maintenance: An Inquiry into Values* (London: Bodley), and Pirsig, R. (1992) *Lila: An Enquiry into Morals* (London: Black Swan).

EXERCISE 1

The historical context of values – poster presentations

This exercise requires a group of at least 10–15 students, but works best with a larger group (40–50 is excellent). If you have a smaller group then you will need to select a range of names and concepts which cover a wide-ranging continuum – for example, from Socrates through to the present day.

The objective is for participants to work in pairs, each pair being given a key thinker or concept specific to the notion of VALUES. They take that name or concept away and 'map' the key thinkers/ideas that have contributed towards our thinking about what has shaped the helping professions as they are today, in the form of a poster presentation.

Students need to be randomly given a name or concept which relates to the exercise – for example, Plato, Thomas Hobbes, R.D. Laing, the civil rights movement, professional codes of practice. They need to then obtain as much information as possible about this person or concept and display it in artistic form on a large A1 poster.

If you are the teacher, lecturer or trainer and have a particular orientation in your teaching (psychology, criminology, nursing etc.) you will need to add names of individuals specific to your profession.

Students should be given at least two to three weeks to prepare their poster and then on the day of presentations all posters need to be put on a 'time continuum' in relation to the historical context of the subject. This creates a very powerful sequencing of ideas in a historical context and helps the students to make links with historical struggles in their profession. This session can take up to three hours to complete (e.g. if you have 50 students each producing one poster each) because all students have to 'visit' each poster. Hence the exercise needs to be structured so that all the students get a chance to ask questions about all the poster topics.

This exercise is exciting and powerful, and rarely fails to exemplify in vivid and dramatic form the development of key thinkers and ideas from the earliest of times to the present day.

The exercise can conclude with a brief presentation by the lecturer/trainer on how our ideas about values now can be traced back in time.

EXERCISE 2

The history of my own value base

This is a complex and challenging exercise for students which is primarily reflective in context (there would be an expectation that students have some understanding of reflective practice). In a sequence of structured exercises, the students explore how their own value base was formed and developed.

SOME ISSUES:

- Because the exercises are very personal, the facilitator assists students in terms of the need to maintain their own boundaries and remain 'grounded'. By grounded, we mean that the student is able to explore issues and will be able to cope with the emotional content. This is not an opportunity for therapy or a 'therapy' group.
- If the session is facilitated, there needs to be clear contracting around the students taking responsibility for self-regulation. At times we can be taken by surprise by 'hidden' feelings, or experiences which we had not fully comprehended. Indeed, some students will be survivors of child abuse, may have experienced recent loss, or find exploring their 'family' or origin overwhelming. *The facilitator should help students to self-monitor and take care when undertaking this exercise. If there are issues that come up, the facilitator should take responsibility for checking the student is OK, and whether they need to just have a breathing space or take time out. Other students should not be drawn into the issues.* Please don't let this put you off what can be a very enriching exercise!

 EXERCISE 3

Orientation

Students should find a photo, object, poem, song, book ... anything that is important to them, and share it with a group of up to five other students. The facilitator should set ground rules where all other students must listen and not interrupt. It's useful for the facilitator to provide an example themselves; here is Jim Wild's, a poem by Jorge Luis Borges, about belonging, and much, much more:

Plainness

The garden's grillwork gate
opens with the ease of a page
in a much-thumbed book,
and, once inside, our eyes
have no need to dwell on objects
already fixed and exact in memory.
Here habits and minds and the private language
all families invent
are everyday things to me.
What necessity is there to speak
or pretend to be someone else?
The whole house knows me,
they're aware of my worries and weaknesses.
This is the best that can happen –
what Heaven perhaps will grant us:
not to be wondered at or required to succeed
but simply to be let in
as a part of an undeniable Reality,
like stones of the road, like trees.

When the students have completed their contributions there should be time for them to share their thoughts in the wider group.

EXERCISE 4

My family of origin and values still retained

The facilitator should assist students in thinking about an important family value from their childhood. This should also be a value that the students still hold central to their lives now. This can be shared with the whole group if they wish. Examples might be 'all people are equal' or 'nuclear war is bad'.

EXERCISE 5

My values unpicked

> The facilitator should help the students to think about a value
> from their childhood which they rejected, and explore what has
> replaced it. This should again be shared with the whole group if
> they wish.

  EXERCISE 6

Mapping out my value base

> The facilitator should direct students to take a large sheet of paper
> and think about it as a map for their values. The centre represents
> 'fundamental' things that they consider will always be a part of
> them. They then map out other issues until they reach the edge
> of the paper where there are words, issues and ideas that are
> vulnerable or not as important. The facilitator could help by
> providing a list that the students use as a primer to expand on.
>   The exercise can last up to 30 minutes. It can be simple, with
> words in one colour, or extensive, with pictures, patterns, quotes
> etc. – the more elaborate versions may require students to work
> on them away from the teaching context before bringing them
> back to share. It's a great exercise to help students really think
> about the issues and experiences that hold our values in place. A
> variation of this is to put around the edge of the paper the things
> that destabilize or threaten our values, which creates some
> interesting points for debate.
>   All these exercises can be designed to act as 'stand alone'
> forms of learning or as part of a module where students can use
> these experiences in an assignment or portfolio. Values are
> fundamental to the development of good practice, but they are
> also constantly challenged by the society we live in and need to
> be re-examined by students and then affirmed throughout an
> individual's career.

chapter **two**

THE SOCIAL WORK VALUE BASE: HUMAN RIGHTS AND SOCIAL JUSTICE IN TALK AND ACTION

Sarah Banks

This chapter explores the concept of a 'value base' for social work. It discusses what we mean by the term, what the core values of social work might be, how they have changed over time and how social workers can live up to their values in the current climate of cost consciousness, performance measurement and marketization of public services. Social work is one of the main 'helping professions', and therefore the professional values developed within it have been influential in, and are broadly similar to, those of other occupational groups in this sector (such as social care work or counselling). This chapter will focus on social work, since it would be too complex to cover each professional/occupational group within the helping professions in such a short space.

Writing and talking about values

I will start by quoting from three professors of social work from the USA and UK who write about social work values (the italics are mine):

> Social work is among *the most value based of all professions* ... Social work's roots are firmly grounded in concepts such as justice and fairness.
>
> (Reamer 1999: 3, 5)

> Social problems and erosion of civic life demand the attention of the profession yet *the social work voice is rarely heard* ... This lack of adherence to the values in the codes is an indicator of the low level of commitment to their importance ...
>
> (Bisman 2004: 110)

> Unequal power relations cut across the emancipatory dimensions of social work values and create oppression through practice ... *Social workers have to become skilful mental acrobats* who can juggle contradictory positions with ease when it comes to putting their values into practice.
>
> (Dominelli 2002: 18)

These quotations all suggest that values are central to social work, but that they are difficult to put into practice. While Reamer's statement may give us a warm glow of satisfaction, conjuring images of social workers as exceptionally committed people of high moral principle, Bisman's comments bring us back to earth with a bump, implying that we do not live up to our fine statements of values and principles. Dominelli expands on this by reminding us of the power of social workers, which means that they can become oppressors themselves, if they are not careful and skilful at handling complexity and contradictions.

I will now quote from some interviews with three senior practitioners in the field of childcare (see Banks 2004 for further details). The interviews were about some of the ethical issues and dilemmas in their work, and the italics here are mine.

> Once you stop putting down *what you think is right for the child* because you can't get that resource, I think we're in a very, very serious situation. Because once you stop recommending it, nobody's ever going to know. So I will always say, this is what should happen.
>
> (Child protection and review manager)

> It's about being very conscious of *the individual needs of the people we're trying to serve*. I would never override the individual needs of a young person or family just because our procedure said that at that point X, Y or Z needed to happen.
>
> (Team manager, childcare)

> What I've spent the last three weeks in, is actually bartering over a residential placement with [placement provider] and saying 'well, if we pay that much more, will you do that much more?' And it's not why I came into social work, I can't believe I'm doing it, and you know, these changes are so insidious really, that you suddenly think, 'what am I doing, talking about *a child's welfare* in terms of how much it's costing?'
>
> (Team manager, child protection)

In these extracts the practitioners are talking about what they believe is right and good in social work practice. They recount some of the struggles in their day-to-day work, using value terms such as: 'right for the child'; 'individual needs'; 'people we are trying to serve'; and 'a child's welfare'. They also speak of their actions – what they tend to do or what they have done – in relation to their values, for example: 'I will always say, this is what should happen'; 'I would never override the individual needs of a young person'; 'bartering over a residential placement'. It is clear from these quotations that the practitioners need not just the skills of mental acrobacy, but a degree of clarity about and commitment to certain values, so they can put them into action. Their comments highlight particular difficulties of implementing values in the prevailing climate of cost-consciousness, privatization and a stress on procedures (Harris 2003; Banks 2004).

The material in the quotations from the professors and professionals gives us more than enough themes to explore in this discussion of values in social work, including:

- What is meant by 'value-based'?
- What are the values of social work?
- Is there a lack of commitment to values on the part of social work practitioners?
- How can social workers live up to their values?

In this chapter, I will say a little more about these questions – but the other chapters that follow will go into more depth in specific areas.

The elusiveness of 'values'

In 1976, a working party on values was set up by the Central Council for Education and Training in Social Work (CCETSW). It produced a discussion paper on *Values in Social Work* (CCETSW 1976). Interestingly, the subheading of the report refers to 'the value bases' (plural) of social work – which hints, perhaps, at some of the difficulties encountered by the group in reaching consensus. In the Introduction, the director of CCETSW, the late Priscilla Young, comments on the complexity of the topic and mentions that the working party encountered problems, including 'argument and dissension' (p. 5). The working party comprised a very distinguished group of theologians, philosophers, sociologists, lecturers in social work/social administration, CCETSW staff and one social worker. Their first problem, it seems, was to define the term 'value'. Some members looked, apparently, to the philosophers in their midst for help, but no help was forthcoming. It is reported that the working party therefore abandoned any attempt to provide a definition in any strict sense.

This difficulty in pinning down a precise meaning for the term 'value' is hardly surprising once we start to reflect on all the possible types of things that might be regarded as 'values' in our ordinary usage of the term – for example, ideologies, attitudes, preferences, beliefs, desires, opinions, the subject matter of which may be moral, cultural, political, religious or aesthetic. Timms (1983: 107), in his classic study of social work values, quotes a literature review that discovered 180 different definitions of the term.

For the purposes of this discussion, however, I will suggest a usage of the term 'values' to mean: particular types of belief that people hold about what is regarded as worthy or valuable. Reference to 'belief' reflects the status that values have in professional life as stronger than mere opinions or preferences. It also reminds us that people *own* values – that is, they are not free-floating statements. We often talk about 'value commitments', which also suggests they may be linked to action.

The social work value base

So, if values are particularly strong kinds of belief, how do we interpret Reamer's statement quoted at the start of this chapter that social work is value-based? Several different types of value may be regarded as fundamental to social work.

Societal values

Social work developed from charitable and philanthropic activities in the latter part of the nineteenth century and grew in the twentieth century as part of state welfare systems premised on values about people's duty to care for one another; the promotion of a more equal distribution of goods; and the enhancement of collective well-being through building individual moral character and self-reliance. In so far as social work maintains a social mandate for the work it does (it is thought to be socially valuable), then it continues to be inextricably linked with prevailing societal values. These values are contested and have changed over time. In the nineteenth century there was a focus on moral welfare and rescue work (much of it quite radical for the time, for example, the work of Josephine Butler rescuing women from a life of prostitution). Charles Loch, of the charity organization Society, writing in 1892, talks about 'the doctrine of the responsibility of charity, as a personal obligation' (Loch 1892: 79). While we may use different language in the twenty-first century in justifying the need for social work and social care, and have moved away from overt paternalism and judgementalism, civic responsibility is still a key theme, along with respect for, and promotion of, human rights, citizen participation, protection of the vulnerable and social inclusion.

Personal values (*including spiritual and political*)

People working in social work and social care are often motivated by their own value commitments. Many of the organizations offering early forms of social work were overtly religious, and some social workers today are inspired by faith or spiritual values. Others have more political motivations based on a desire to change social structures, and challenge inequality and oppression. Many simply express a 'desire to help people' or 'to give something back'. In common with other practitioners in welfare, caring and social action work, the values that social workers bring to their work and develop and form during the course of their practice are an integral part of what we mean by the 'value base' of the work.

Professional values

As social work became professionalized in the twentieth century, explicit statements of shared values were produced. We find written statements of values in textbooks, guidelines for education and training, and codes of ethics or conduct. They reflect the social and political climates of the places and times where they were written and the motivations and commitments of the current and past members of the occupational group of social work. They are also designed to influence and challenge prevailing societal norms and values and to develop, enhance or define the value commitments of individual practitioners. In this sense, they can be seen as a meeting point for societal and personal values. The values included, and their definitions, vary. At a very general level there is some consensus, as exemplified in a statement of ethical principles from the International Federation of Social Workers (IFSW) (2004). This is based on two sets of core values:

1 *Human rights and dignity* – the promotion of and respect for people's rights to choice; encouraging participation in decision-making; treating each person as a whole; promoting empowerment based on strengths.

2 *Social justice* – challenging negative discrimir
policies and practices; recognizing diversity; d
sources fairly according to need; working in sol

A third element is entitled 'professional conduct' and covers specific principles relating to the professional role, including maintaining the competence to do the job, confidentiality in the professional relationship and acting with 'compassion, empathy and care'. The statement produced by the IFSW is inevitably rather generic, as it aims to be relevant to social work around the world. In one sense the IFSW is a cross between an international grouping of professional associations and a global social movement with a specific focus on social justice.

National codes of ethics are often more detailed, with a greater focus on professional identity and roles. One example is the code of ethics of the British Association of Social Workers (BASW) (2002), which draws on the very similar statements produced by professional associations in the USA (National Association of Social Workers – NASW – 1999) and Australia (Australian Association of Social Workers – AASW – 2000). In addition to the values of respect for and promotion of human rights, dignity and social justice, it includes 'service' – the utilitarian ideal of promoting welfare or well-being combined with the altruistic idea of serving humanity; 'integrity', which could be regarded as a quality of character; and 'competence', an ability and commitment to practise proficiently. I have summarized the values in the BASW code as follows:

1 *Respect for the dignity and worth of all human beings* – in the context of social work, this applies particularly to service users, and includes respecting and promoting individuals' and groups' rights to self-determination.
2 *Promotion of social justice* – this includes working to remove inequalities and promoting fair distribution of goods and services among people and groups.
3 *Service to humanity* – the promotion of welfare or well-being of service users and in society generally.
4 *Integrity* – upholding the values and standards of the profession, including honesty, reliability and impartiality.
5 *Competence* – proficiency in practice, developing knowledge and skills and using expertise in development of welfare policies and programmes.

e these statements of values enough?

In social work, as in many other professions, we are very good at producing lists of values – and indeed we are getting better and better at it. We tend to turn to statements of professional values, particularly those in codes of ethics, when talking about the 'value base' of social work. Such statements have both strengths and weaknesses. Some of the weaknesses are summarized below.

- *Abstraction* – value statements such as those listed above are often criticized as too abstract, as being divorced from the social and political contexts of the work. This may encourage us to see professional values as somehow living a life of their own – forgetting their intimate relationship with prevailing societal values and our own personal values, and the potential for conflict and contradiction. The creation of such lists of values also involves an artificial separation of values from knowledge and skills, and from the realities of everyday practice. We need to remember that the values of social work do not exist in isolation from the societies and cultures in which they are practised, nor from the employing organizations, practitioners and service users involved.
- *Western orientation* – value statements have also been criticized as being too western in outlook, especially in their focus on human rights. Within the concept of 'human rights' there may be a conflict between the rights of individuals and the rights of peoples – cultural or religious groupings. The stress on rights to privacy and confidentiality is premised on a western concept of the freely choosing individual person, whereas in many countries and cultures the extended family group or community is regarded as the basic unit.
- *Open to interpretation* – the values are expressed very generally and are open to wide interpretation. The concept of 'social justice', for example, may be partly defined in terms of promoting a fair distribution of resources. But what counts as 'fair' may vary according to need, merit and so forth.
- *Implementation gap* – even if we have broad agreement about what the values mean, there is no guarantee that people can or will put them into practice.
- *Devised by professionals/professional bodies* – the sets of values in the codes of ethics tend to be devised by groups of professionals. They may not necessarily reflect the values of

service users, carers or the public generally. The language is often relatively inaccessible – abstract, general and profession-alized.

There are, however, some positive roles played by such lists of values, which include:

- *Drawing attention to the gap between rhetoric and reality* – although we may condemn the artificiality of separating values from knowledge and skills, and all three from the realities of everyday practice, the exercise of so doing, and then studying them in our laboratories – lecture rooms, councils and committees – may serve a useful purpose in drawing our attention to lapses, lack of clarity, inconsistencies and, above all, gaps between our rhetorical words and our practical actions.
- *Contributing to professional identity and integrity* – the idea of a distinctive social work professional identity may or may not be regarded as a good thing – especially in a climate of increasing interprofessional working. A list of values can serve as a constant reminder of the kinds of people social workers should be and how they should act. If there is a clear statement of values to which workers are committed, then it may encourage them to act with integrity (consistency and coherence), especially when under pressure to conform to performance targets or inappropriate procedures (as the quo-tations from the social workers given earlier demonstrate).
- *Can serve as a focus for resistance to inhumane and unjust policies and practices* – this follows on from the point above. A sense of sharing and holding on to a set of collective values to which one is also personally committed can be helpful and, indeed, may be vital, in combating injustice and oppression, and working for change at a policy and political level.

We may conclude that statements of professional values do serve a purpose, although they need to be viewed with caution. They are a starting point for an ongoing dialogue about values in practice. But we need to broaden out the dialogue to include service users, the general public, politicians and policy-makers in order to open up the discussion and debate. It is important that we do not allow professional values to become divorced from their societal context or, indeed, from our own personal respon-sibility and ownership. Professional values should, in fact, be an ongoing dialogue between societal values and social workers' own personal values and motivations (which include emotional and political dimensions).

Concluding comments: reaffirming our value base

To conclude this chapter, I will summarize two important themes that have emerged from the discussion, which are about ways of looking at values.

First, *values as commitments with societal, professional and personal (emotional and political) dimensions.* We can regard social work as a job (working for an employer doing a specific set of tasks in a particular setting), a profession (belonging to a community of practitioners sharing knowledge and values), a vocation (a calling to do good in the world) and a social movement (campaigning and working for change on issues of poverty and injustice). 'Vocation' and 'social movement' imply a stronger and deeper commitment to the process and the ends of the work. Such values are built on relationships of care and compassion between people, as well as a more global concern for the achievement of greater equality in the allocation of social goods between nations, communities and individuals. Vocation and social movement go beyond the demands of job and profession, as narrowly conceived. These elements have always been present in social work, but they do not sit very easily in the current context of marketization and managerialism.

Second, *values at the heart of social work practice – reasserting the emotional and political dimensions.* Many commentators, such as Cynthia Bisman (2004), whom I quoted at the start of this chapter, have castigated social work for its fine rhetoric about a solid and firm value base, while failing to live up to its stated commitment to social justice. It may be more useful to talk not about a value base (which implies something solid serving as a foundation) but rather about values as the core, indeed the heart, of our practice, as Bisman recommends. This then allows the values to be fluid and shifting, but suggests that they belong to us, and we must therefore recognize, question and nurture them collectively – as workers, service users, carers, volunteers, employers, educators and policy-makers.

Bernard Bosanquet wrote an article in the *Charity Organisation Review* of 1898 entitled 'Idealism in social work'. He suggests that idealism has two sides: passion and logic. He refers to Plato's description of the genuine idealist, who has faith in the good purpose of the world, and is spurred by the passion and the logic of reality. At the time of Bosanquet's writing we can probably think of several people in the field who were spurred on by passion and logic – such as Octavia Hill in her pioneering and meticulous work on social housing (Young and Ashton 1956: 115–25), Augustus Barnett, involved in founding of Toynbee Hall, the university settlement in East London (Picht 1914) and Jane Addams, who developed Hull House, the first settlement in America (Addams 1910).

Today, in the midst of the perverse logic of markets, managerialism and measurement – the kind of climate referred to by the three childcare practitioners quoted earlier – it may seem hard for passion to win through. But it is still there. We can look to many of the people writing chapters in this book to inspire us as role models, and we can look to each other for collective dialogue and solidarity.

I am sure the rest of the chapters in this book will take us further with the concept of passion – which is, I think, an important component of living social work values, related to compassion, anger at injustice and above all, a commitment to action.

References

Addams, J. (1910) *Twenty Years at Hull House,* with autobiographical notes. New York: Macmillan.

Australian Association of Social Workers (AASW) (2000) *AASW Code of Ethics*. Kingston: AASW.

Banks, S. (2004) *Ethics, Accountability and the Social Professions*. Basingstoke: Palgrave Macmillan.

Bisman, C. (2004) Social work values: the moral core of the profession, *British Journal of Social Work*, 34: 109–23.

Bosanquet, B. (1898) Idealism in social work, *Charity Organisation Review*, 3(March): 122–33.

British Association of Social Workers (BASW) (2002) *The Code of Ethics for Social Work*. Birmingham: BASW.

CCETSW (Central Council for Education and Training in Social Work) (1976) *Values in Social Work: A Discussion Paper Produced by the Working Party on the Teaching of the Value Bases of Social Work*. London: CCETSW.

Dominelli, L. (2002) Values in social work, in R. Adams, L. Dominelli and M. Payne (eds) *Critical Practice in Social Work*, pp. 15–27. Basingstoke: Palgrave Macmillan.

Harris, J. (2003) *The Social Work Business*. London: Routledge.

International Federation of Social Workers (IFSW) and International Association of Schools of Social Work (IASSW) (2004) *Ethics in Social Work, Statement of Principles*. Berne: IFSW and IASSW.

Loch, C. (1892) *Charity Organisation*. London: Swan Sonnenschein & Co.

National Association of Social Workers (NASW) (1999) *Code of Ethics*. Washington: NASW.

Picht, W. (1914) *Toynbee Hall and the English Settlement Movement*. London: G. Bell & Sons.

Reamer, F. (1999) *Social Work Values and Ethics*, 2nd edn. New York: Columbia University Press.

Young, A. and Ashton, E. (1956) *British Social Work in the Nineteenth Century*. London: Routledge & Kegan Paul.

Further reading

Banks, S. (2001) Professional values in informal education work, in L. Richardson and M. Wolfe (eds) *Principles and Practice of Informal Education: Learning through life*, pp. 62–73. London: Routledge.

Banks, S. (2006) *Ethics and Values in Social Work*, 3rd edn. Basingstoke: Palgrave Macmillan.

Bond, T. (2000) *Standards and Ethics for Counselling in Action*, 2nd edn. London: Sage.

General Social Care Council (GSCC) (2002) *Codes of Practice for Social Care Workers and Employers*. London: GSCC.

Tjeltveit, A. (1999) *Ethics and Values in Psychotherapy*. London: Routledge.

The following exercises will explore some of the dilemmas raised by Sarah Banks. These are best done in small groups with a facilitator, but can be adapted for self-directed work, distance learning or e-based learning. Students can work through them alone if necessary.

 ## EXERCISE 1

The value base of social work and social care

The facilitator should direct students to form small groups to discuss and document the following questions arising from Sarah's chapter for about 15 minutes before reporting back. The facilitator should document key points from each group.

1   What is meant by 'value-based'?
2   What are the values of social work?
3   Is there a lack of commitment to values on the part of social work practitioners?
4   How can social workers live up to their values?

 ## EXERCISE 2

The realities of practice?

In this exercise students are asked to focus on the 'realities' of practice, again in small groups. The idea is that each group should explore the history and emergence of such issues as 'best value', 'modernization' and the role of the private sector in social work and social care services.

In her chapter, Sarah Banks provides examples from practice where workers felt their values were compromised:

> Once you stop putting down *what you think is right for the child* because you can't get that resource, I think we're in a very, very serious situation. Because once you stop recommending it, nobody's ever going to know. So I will always say, this is what should happen.
>
> (Child protection and review manager)

It's about being very conscious of *the individual needs of the people we're trying to serve*. I would never override the individual needs of a young person or family just because our procedure said that at that point X, Y or Z needed to happen.

(Team manager, childcare)

What I've spent the last three weeks in, is actually bartering over a residential placement with [placement provider] and saying 'well, if we pay that much more, will you do that much more?' And it's not why I came into social work, I can't believe I'm doing it, and you know, these changes are so insidious really, that you suddenly think, 'what am I doing, talking about *a child's welfare* in terms of how much it's costing?'

(Team manager, child protection)

The facilitator should ask each group to consider the following policy concepts and suggest what they might mean. Allow about ten minutes on each before allowing the students to give their feedback and then moving on to the second part of the exercise.

Part 1

1   Best Value
2   Modernization
3   'Mixed economy'
4   Contracting out services

Part 2

1   Can you put a price on helping relationships?
2   Should helping others be a source of money-making?
3   Are helping services 'finite' in terms of resources?
4   Who should make the decisions about who provides resources?

The above issues provide a great opportunity for students to think about critical issues which relate to values. This could then be developed into a debate with managers who are part of the 'contract culture'. They could be invited to take part in a debate on the subject the following week.

chapter **three**

GLOBALIZATION DEFINED

George Ritzer and Adam Barnard

Children as young as 2 recognize the golden arches of McDonald's. Starbucks, Disney, Nike and Adidas have become global brands that are instantly recognizable and have permeated every high street and home. The Nike 'swooshstika' is reportedly the most requested tattoo in North America (Klein 2004). Political events from around the world are reported immediately, such as 9/11 or the Asian tsunami. We mostly use Microsoft software on computers and are likely to have shopped in a Wal-Mart-owned store. What does this tell us? Clearly, a process of globalization has led to distinct changes in our everyday lives. Drugs, crime, sex, war, protest, terrorism, disease, people, ideas, images, news, information, entertainment, pollution, goods and money all travel the globe (Held 2004).

In terms of culture (Hopper 2007), society (Barnett *et al.* 2005), politics (Bayart 2007) and economics (Kaplinsky 2005; Held and Kaya 2006), rapid and dramatic change has taken place due to globalization. Wikipedia – a good example of this process – suggests that globalization refers to increasing global connectivity, integration and interdependence in the economic, social, technological, cultural, political and ecological spheres.

What does this suggest to us about the contemporary world? How are we to understand this process? What does it mean for globalized communities? What challenges and opportunities does it raise for the social care and helping professions in the twenty-first century?

The dimensions of globalization

There is no question that the world is currently undergoing significant and profound acceleration in the process of globalization, but globalization itself is not new. For example, trade has existed for millennia between areas such as the Roman Empire, Arabia and China. Knowledge, science, technology and culture have always been global throughout history. However, many commentators suggest that we are now witnessing a qualitatively different set of processes which seem unchangeable.

Globalization achieved unprecedented heights in the last half of the twentieth century and has accelerated further in the early twenty-first century. That dramatic growth has led to much work in many different fields on the topic of globalization and many efforts have been made to define it. Held (2004) suggests globalization involves four dimensions. The first is the *stretching of social relations* so that cultural, economic and political networks are connected across the world. For example, different and dispersed communities are part of global 'diasporas' of peoples spread beyond any nation or locality, so that communities are constituted across territorial boundaries.

The second dimension is an *intensification of flows of interaction* so that instant communication is available to many (if you have access to the mass media, TV, internet or telephone). Trade and commerce, entertainment, news and media, sport, art and culture are all experienced rapidly and in a far greater volume than before.

The third dimension is the *increasing interpenetration of distant cultures and events* as societies come face to face with each other. For example, Bollywood films, the diversity of food available and the global recognition of brands such as Coke, Disney, Microsoft and McDonald's. The tragedy that occurred on 9/11 shows how we are influenced and affected by geographically distant and remote events.

Finally, the fourth dimension is the *emergence of global infrastructures* to support and drive these changes. The internet is often identified as a key emerging infrastructure that supports stretched social relations, encourages intensified communication and brings people and places closer together, although in an uneven and divided way (Drori 2006). So how might we summarize these changes and processes?

Towards a definition

Ritzer defines globalization as 'an accelerating set of processes involving flows that encompass ever-greater numbers of the world's spaces and that lead to increasing integration and interconnectivity among those spaces' (2004: 72). Giddens (2002) refers to these processes as a 'runaway world' and Marshal McLuhan (McLuhan and Powers 1989) speaks of the 'global village'. Woodward (2003: 171) suggests globalization is:

A social, cultural, political and economic phenomenon, which is subject to many different interpretations, ranging from those who see its impact as minimal and nothing new, to globalists or globalizers who argue that it is a recent and very significant phenomenon which has transformed life across the world. Some read this as a positive experience whilst others see it as having disastrous effects on local communities and those outside the western, especially US, mainstream. Most commentators agree that it has had some transforming impact.

Globalization transforms our everyday lives, from minor considerations of what to have for dinner to major world-changing events. It involves social, economic, political, cultural and environmental processes and is characterized by conflict (such as terrorism and war) as well as consensus (such as communication and entertainment). It is also characterized by a crossing of boundaries of nation states (Woodward 2003: 137). Events in one country are no longer isolated, such as the fall of the Berlin Wall, pollution or natural disasters. All have far-reaching effects that are transnational and global.

Globalization is divided between winners and losers. 'Positive globalizers' see everyone benefiting from the expansion of globalization, while 'negative globalizers' see losers missing out on the benefits and suffering increased exploitation. Global networks and flows operate differently for different groups of people and communities. Debates concerning 'race' and gender, so often central to social care, have been subsumed or marginalized in the mainstream of globalization (Adam 2002). For example, Saskia Sassen (1998) argues than in global cities (such as London, Tokyo and New York), most of the daily servicing jobs are carried out by women, immigrants and people from minority ethnic groups (often the same person).

Globalization allegedly presents opportunities of greater democracy and participation, such as through the internet, but this technology remains dominated by the wealthy areas of the world. There is fast transmission of information, easy access for individuals and communities and new opportunities for ideas, markets, democracy and choice. However, speed is of more importance to rich nations and it is this very speed that leads us into a rapid and manic sense of consciousness where we often fail to reflect on the consequences of our actions. Ideas can be censured, choice is restricted to global brands and products, and democracy can be blocked, stifled or monitored. Globalization has allowed easier movement of people across the globe but migration is often prevented for many refugees and migrants. Globalization is often economically driven, and exploitation remains and deepens.

Globalization and communities

Let us consider just a few examples of money, communication, 'sameness' (homogeneity) and consumption, with special emphasis on their impact on community (the discussion that follows draws heavily on Appadurai's 1996 work, *Modernity at Large*, and his sense of global 'scapes'). Vast sums of money circulate around the world through government treasuries, banks, brokerage houses and so on. However, most of this flow is largely invisible to us, although it can have a profound effect on our lives. The focus throughout this chapter is the impact of globalization on communities, so how do global flows of money affect them? In many ways, of course, but one of the most important occurs when global traders in money decide that the currency of a given nation is overvalued. The result is a decline in the value of that currency with devastating effects on whole societies (e.g. several East Asian countries in 1997; Argentina in 2002). Buying power declines as local currencies are devalued. Jobs are lost and increasing numbers find themselves out of work and short of money. The community suffers in various ways without any control over the process.

Let us also consider communication. Some commentators have suggested the world has become 'flat' (Friedman 2005) due to horizontal and less hierarchical forms of communication, such as the internet, and it is certainly true that a far wider range of people are now able to communicate their views and get their message across. We are now made aware of the struggle for democracy in China, the living conditions for the people of Iraq and popular protests in South America. This can have a salutary effect on communities which are able to get their views out and to have them reaffirmed by others scattered throughout the world. That said, the reverse is the case because those who seek to destroy a community can use the same media to organize and carry out their destructive activities (e.g. censorship in China). Terrorism, crime and drugs have all benefited from globalization. Hence, the world has not become anything approaching flat as inequality and exploitation remain rife.

A major issue is the degree to which globalization is related to a growing homogeneity (becoming the same or 'sameness'), or a sustained heterogeneity (being diverse and different) (Ritzer 2004, 2005). This has great implications for communities since the latter would imply the continued survival and vitality of diverse and distinct communities while the former involves a loss of distinctiveness, with diverse communities becoming more and more alike.

'McDonaldization' is the process by which the principles of the fast food restaurant are affecting more and more sectors of society, and an increasing number of societies around the world (Ritzer 2004). The idea that more and more societies are being affected by and are adopting the *same* principles (e.g. efficiency) means that 'McDonaldization' tends to be associated with increasing homogenization. At a most basic level, many communities around the world look increasingly alike because so many of them have one, or more, McDonald's restaurants (there are over 30,000 of them, most outside the USA), to say nothing of many of McDonald's clones in the fast food business (e.g. Burger King, KFC etc.). More generally, more and more organizations operate on basically the same principles, so we can talk about things like 'McUniversities', 'McDoctors' and 'McPharmacies'.

As powerful as the process of 'McDonaldization' may be, we are still a long way from completely homogeneous communities and the eradication of diversity. Much remains different about communities from one area of a given nation to another, to say nothing of one part of the world to another. Furthermore, 'McDonaldization' has resulted in a counter-reaction that has led to more, rather than less, diversity. Individuals, groups, communities and even large, global organizations such as Slow Food, based in Italy, have mounted significant opposition to McDonald's and 'McDonaldization'. Slow Food is particularly important in this regard for its defence of distinctive cities ('Slow Cities'), local communities, and traditional food and other products. For example, in his defence of locally-produced food, José Bové, a modest agricultural farmer, has become an international icon of resistance to global capitalism (Bové and Dufour 2005).

However, there is a deeper kind of homogeneity in the sense that people become ever more deeply enmeshed in consumer culture. This means that consumption becomes increasingly important to them, and a primary focus of their lives. We can enjoy sun-dried Italian tomatoes while drinking American coke on Ikea settees watching *Big Brother*. There is a threat to heterogeneity when local, diverse products and practices are eroded by a global consumer culture. Would you rather have cheap standardized shoes made in sweat-shop conditions in a distant country by child labour or a bespoke pair of handmade shoes made by a local artisan? If the global economy had not made the former so cheap, we might all prefer the latter.

Those who want to sustain communities and their diversity will want to oppose much of what is described above. Heterogeneity at many levels is what makes life and communities interesting and rewarding, and importantly, as part of the process of homogenization, control shifts from inside a community to outside it, giving external forces the capacity to alter or even destroy that community (large superstores, supermarkets and shopping centres are a good example in certain cases). Such organizations are essentially in the business of making money and very often they do so by exploiting communities and their people, as well as by taking profits to another community, perhaps even to another nation (Klein 2004). All of this can leave a community greatly impoverished, economically, politically and culturally.

However, we must not forget that globalization is *not* a one-way street; a unidimensional process. Just as many things flow into any given community, many things also flow out. Globalization can have many positive effects on many things, including communities. Many communities have been greatly enhanced by the arrival of global businesses, the global media, global sports teams and the like. In assessing the impact of globalization we need to look at both a community's gains and losses. Positive commentators have suggested that it is not clear that anything needs to be done about globalization in general, but it is clear that communities need to seek out that which enhances them and to block that which threatens them and their integrity, or to limit the impact of what cannot be blocked.

The future, social care and the helping professions

What of the future? It seems clear that globalization is here to stay and the future will bring only an acceleration of it and its effects on everything, including communities. There will certainly continue to be many positives associated with this process, but it is also the case that the negative effects will continue. The thrust of this discussion leads us to a concern that the negatives will come to outweigh the positives. After all, the greater power and a disproportionate share of wealth are held by the forces that support 'McDonaldization', consumerism and homogeneity. In confrontations with most communities, they have the upper hand (although there are certainly instances where the community 'David' has slain the corporate 'Goliath'). Thus, it is hard to envision a bright future for communities, at least as we have traditionally thought of them. A highly 'McDonaldized' community, one in which much of what transpires is centrally conceived and controlled, is a long way from what we have thought of (perhaps over-romantically) as 'community'. We will need to rethink what we mean by 'community', but this is far less of a problem than being forced to abandon communities to the larger forces that seek to eviscerate them and to profit from denuding them of what makes them unique and special.

There can be distinctly advantageous byproducts of globalization: the sharing of customs, traditions, ways of life, increased variety and richness in culture, entertainment, sport and the arts, and breaking down territorial boundaries and insular mentalities. It can give us a vibrant, diverse, dynamic and independent culture that draws from a multitude of sources. On the other hand, globalization can produce a homogenized culture. Cities appear the same, with uniform chain stores, global brands and supermarkets seated in a lifeless, static, consumer culture imposed by corporations.

For social care and the helping services, both positive and negative globalization presents a huge range of challenges. For example, child protection issues are now global concerns with trafficking, exploitation, sex tourism and abuse increasingly coordinated across national boundaries. Adult care services need to account for and be mindful of global dimensions to care, such as respecting and valuing the diversity of peoples and cultures, and respecting links to geographically distant communities. However, few commentators have focused on how globalization has impacted on social care practice. Dominelli and Hoogvelt (1996) demonstrate the significance of globalization on the process of intervention in social care. As a result of global market forces, needs-led assessments and relationship-building have given way to budget-led assessments, increased managerial control over practitioners and bureaucratized procedures for handling consumer complaints. Social care has tended to be re-orientated away from its commitment to holistic provision and social justice and towards homogenized and bureaucratic responses. Globalization adds to the pressure for health and social care to abandon its historic mission to promote equality and social justice. It can also accelerate the breakdown of communities and lead to aggravated social problems among marginalized and excluded groups.

Dominelli (2007) explores the opportunities and constraints that the dynamics of globalization present for human development in a range of different countries and situations. Arguing that

globalization is currently a system of organizing social rela
along neo-liberal lines, Dominelli examines practical example
how people respond to significant social changes in their communities. Globalization has collapsed the boundaries of time, space
and place in ways that have exacerbated inequality, at the same
time giving rise to unparalleled riches for some and the illusion of
equality for all (after all, everyone can commune with a Big Mac).

The skill of the globalized worker is to retain the humanity,
holism, justice and opportunities that globalization can bring,
while protecting communities from exploitation and inequality.
Beckett and Maynard (2005) suggest that social work, and the
helping professions generally, deal with people who in one way of
other are marked as different and to various degrees excluded
from mainstream society. The challenge for social work and the
helping professions is therefore to operate in a way which as far
as possible challenges and reduces that exclusion, rather than
confirming and legitimizing it. In a 'globalized' world this challenge is ever more important and central to social work, social
care and the helping professions.

References

Adam, B. (2002) The gendered time politics of globalization: of shadow-
lands and elusive justice, *Feminist Review*, 70: 3–29.

Appadurai, A. (1996) *Modernity at Large: Cultural Dimensions of Globalization*. Minneapolis, MN: University of Minnesota Press.

Barnett, A., Held, D. and Henderson, C. (2005) *Debating Globalization*.
Cambridge: Polity Press.

Bayart, F. (2007) *Governance of the World*. Cambridge: Polity Press.

Beckett, C. and Maynard, A. (2005) *Values and Ethics in Social Work: An
Introduction*. London: Sage.

Bové, J. and Dufour, F. (2005) *Food for the Future: Agriculture for a Global
Age*. Cambridge: Polity Press.

Dominelli, L. (2007) (ed.) *Revitalising Communities in a Globalising World*.
London: Ashgate.

Dominelli, L. and Hoogvelt, A. (1996) Globalization and the technocra-
tization of social work, *Critical Social Policy*, 16(47): 45–62.

Drori, G. (2006) *Global E-Litism: Digital Inequality, Social Inequality, and
Transnationality*. New York: Worth.

Friedman, T. (2005) *The World is Flat: A Brief History of the Twenty-First
Century*. New York: Farrar, Straus & Giroux.

Giddens, A. (2002) *Runaway World: The Reith lectures*, 2nd edn. London:
Profile Books.

Held. D. (2004) *A Globalising World?: Culture, Economics, Politics*, 2nd edn.
Maidenhead: Open University Press.

Held, D. and Kaya, A. (2006) *Global Inequality: A Comprehensive Introduction*. Cambridge: Polity Press.

Hopper, P. (2007) *Understanding Cultural Globalization*. Cambridge: Polity Press.

Kaplinsky, R. (2005) *Globalization, Poverty and Inequality: Between a Rock and a Hard Place*. Cambridge: Polity Press.

Klein, N. (2004) *No Logo; No Space, No Jobs, No Choice; Taking Aim at the Brand Bullies*. London: Flamingo.

McLuhan, M. and Powers, B.R. (1989) *The Global Village: Transformations in World Life and Media in the 21st Century*. Oxford: Oxford University Press.

Ritzer, G. (2004) *The McDonaldization of Society*. Revised New Century Edition. Thousand Oaks, CA: Pine Forge Press.

Ritzer, G. (2005) *Enchanting a Disenchanted World: Revolutionizing the Means of Consumption*. Thousand Oaks, CA: Pine Forge Press.

Sassen, S. (1998) *Globalization and the Discontents: Essays on the New Mobilities of People and Money*. New York: The New Press.

Woodward, K. (2003) *Social Sciences: the Big Issues*. Maidenhead: Open University Press.

EXERCISE 1

Business, money and local communities

Think about George Ritzer's comment earlier in this chapter:

> The focus throughout this chapter is the impact of globalization on communities, so how do global flows of money affect them? In many ways, of course, but one of the most important occurs when global traders in money decide that the currency of a given nation is overvalued. The result is a decline in the value of that currency with devastating effects on whole societies (e.g. several East Asian countries in 1997; Argentina in 2002). Buying power declines as local currencies are devalued. Jobs are lost and increasing numbers find themselves out of work and short of money. The community suffers in various ways ...

Before carrying out the exercise, one of the following films should be shown to the group: *Roger & Me* or *The Big One* by Michael Moore. Both films explore the devastation of local communities when multinational companies 'relocate' or 'downsize' to other less developed countries in the world where wages are less. In both films Moore attempts to talk with those who made the decisions that affected local communities. These films can be purchased at most outlets which sell back copies of old films and are easily located on the internet.

The facilitator should then request students to form into small groups and carry out the following task.

Through discussion in your group identify a local community which was once thriving (e.g. a mining community, a particular manufacturing base such as steel). Explore the reasons why that community collapsed. If possible, interview people who were once part of that community. Find out about:

- The community at its height
- Why that industry collapsed – what were the reasons given at the time?
- Where in the world is that industry now thriving?
- What happened when the industry collapsed?
- What happened to the community?
- How robust is the community now?
- How long did it take for the community to recover?

Much of the information you obtain will be from individual testimonies and biographical details from those 'looking back'. Care and sensitivity should be shown when interviewing individuals who experienced personal distress and anguish.

EXERCISE 2

Globalized companies and the products you purchase

Many of us buy goods and services from companies identified as a 'global' brand. However, we rarely consider who made those goods, how much they were paid, the conditions they work in and whether we would feel anxious about the purchase if we knew more. This was made shockingly clear to Jim Wild (one of the editors of this book) when he went to purchase what he though was a locally made wardrobe. When he spoke to the assistant he discovered that the item he wanted was imported from China. The local company in Sheffield sent the wood for the wardrobe out to China and it was then delivered back to the 'local' shop. The owner did not know what wages were paid or the conditions for the workers and said he did not want to know.

Ask students to go to a shop which is a national brand, find something that is made in one of the new emerging economies (China or India) and ask whether there is an ethical policy in place.

Alternative exercise

1 Get students into small groups of six to eight people.
2 Ask them to draw up a list of all the items the students are wearing that are global brands (e.g. Nike, Adidas).
3 Each person should then find out where the item was manufactured.
4 Each person should then find out what the conditions were like for those individuals who produced that item. There are pressure groups in the 'fair trade' world who can help, but asking the companies directly would be interesting in that they will almost certainly not want to reveal the true facts about what they are paying their employees.

EXERCISE 3

My town is like your town

Consider the following quote from earlier in the chapter:

> there is a deeper kind of homogeneity in the sense that people become ever more deeply enmeshed in consumer culture. This means that consumption becomes increasingly important to them, and a primary focus of their lives.

After reading this quote, ask students to audit the shopping facilities in their town. The facilitator should divide them into groups so that they do not duplicate each other's work. They should make a list of the 'top ten' shops and then compare them with the other groups' lists.

 EXERCISE 4

Consumer culture

The following people have said a great deal about 'consumer culture' and how such a rampant pursuit of materialism will have a bad effect on our development as human beings. Students should produce a one-page summary of the beliefs of one of the people listed below. Some support consumption, and others are against it.

- Eric Fromm
- Herbert Marcuse
- Karl Marx
- Thorsten Veblen
- Naomi Klein
- Guy Debord
- Jean Baudrillard
- Oliver James

Chapter **four**

AN ANTI-RACIST STRATEGY FOR INDIVIDUAL AND ORGANIZATIONAL CHANGE

Beth E. Richie

I have framed this chapter to complement the other contributors to this volume and to encourage practitioners, scholars, activists and writers to reaffirm radical social work values in the interest of social transformation and social change. I begin by revealing key assumptions about racism, inequality and power as they shape social arrangements in contemporary society. I then define some of the concepts that I think are most useful in reframing the work before turning attention to concrete strategies for engaging in radical anti-racist praxis and building relationships with activist allies. The final part of the chapter will focus on long-term strategies for change.

The problems with 'individually-focused' social work practice

I draw my critique of individually-focused social work practice from my professional training as a social worker and my work in a community-based human service agency in an all black community in New York City for a number of years. My work focused on reproductive justice, gender violence, incarceration, issues of sexuality and the problem of state violence towards institutionalized and other vulnerable groups of black women. I worked in prisons with battered women, in juvenile detention centres with girls who identified as lesbians, with prostitutes who are assaulted by both police officers and their customers, and with women who are poor, addicted to drugs and otherwise in compromised positions in contemporary society. I came to understand my roles as a social worker as:

1   Responding to the immediate crisis of abuse, poverty, harassment or incarceration.
2   Helping my clients (prostitutes, battered women, prisoners and others) to navigate the dangers associated with institutionalization.
3   Working with those in trouble to find the support and resources they need to heal.

Despite the fact that these were noble goals, they are totally insufficient to my current understanding of what constitutes good social work intervention. In my view it is not good enough to keep developing more services – even if they are good services – and provide them in greater doses to those who are most disadvantaged in our society. In fact, a practice that merely offers services as people's troubles mount could, by some measures, be considered irresponsible.

Put another way, an ethic of social work that is committed to social justice would consider that working only on individual cases to help prostitutes get charges brought against them dropped – *while ignoring the factors that led them to become involved in sex work in the first place* — as wholly insufficient. Similarly, helping battered women to get an order of protection from law enforcement agencies after a violent assault – *without attending to their long-term needs for safety* – is counter to the type of intervention that will lead to societal transformation. Furthermore, only helping women in prison get early parole – *without ensuring that they have a place to live* – or working to ensure that girls in lock-down get to go to school while they are in detention – *without providing for their ongoing educational, health or economic needs* – is, from some vantage points, equally irresponsible.

In this chapter, I am arguing that when social workers only respond to the immediate crisis situations affecting the vulnerable people with whom they engage, then professional intervention can have a harmful effect because 'making it better on the individual level in a crisis' means that the lives of people with problems become decontextualized. The complexity of their situation is reduced to their specific problem. When this happens, social workers only need to take responsibility for providing immediate care, as opposed to looking towards the overall well-being of a person, a family or a community. It becomes possible to treat symptoms rather than root causes of problems. In times of conservative politics, it becomes easy to assign blame for individual problems to individual people, rather than looking at the position that people are in, and their subsequent limited access to opportunity.

It is important for social workers to move beyond an individual analysis of social problems in order for real social change to occur. Undoubtedly, providing shelter to battered women saves their lives (Bennett *et al.* 2004). However, as currently operated, such refuges also remove women from their communities and absolve those communities of their responsibility to provide safety and protection. In addition, when such shelters are operated by professionals, there is an assumption that replacing abusive men's authority over women's lives with a social worker's authority is a good thing, which patently it is not.

Another example can be found in the work on behalf of girls in detention. Many professionals argue for more counselling and more 'gender-specific' programmes (Goodkind 2005). In so doing, what they are saying is that girls in lock-down deserve better services, which is true. But this argument fails to recognize that if offering programmes becomes the only or the primary goal, it distracts attention from the problems that lead to girls being arrested in the first place. It does little to challenge the overall repressive tendencies of the criminal legal system (Herivel and Wright 2003).

From individual analyses to organizational change

As implied by the title of this chapter, moving beyond an individual analysis requires that social workers attend to issues of organizational and societal change. In my view, social workers have resisted this move in great part because we have divested a critical analysis of power from the values that guide our practice (Franklin 2001; Gambrill 2001). This has created a fundamental flaw in our work which is rendered ineffective at getting to the root causes of social problems. Decidedly apolitical, social work practice has become invested in a rhetorical, charity-oriented approach to social care rather than being a radical approach to social transformation. A pivotal aspect of this lack of critical analysis is the silence we assume about issues of race and structural racism in our practice.

Issues of institutionalized racism, and the subsequent social inequality based on ethnicity, powerfully organize social arrangements in contemporary society. As a result, 'communities of colour' globally face disproportionate disadvantage on most measures of social well-being. These disadvantages are concentrated, persistent and increasingly considered inevitable consequences of a multicultural society where the goal of superficial integration supersedes the goal of true social equality. As a result, conservative analyses of problems (including health disparities, disproportionate rates of incarceration and multigenerational poverty) are understood to be evidence of so-called 'community disorganization', 'social deviance', 'family breakdown' or 'individual immorality', as opposed to issues of abuses of power and injustice.

It is important to emphasize that this conceptualization is deeply ideological. Indeed, the ways of understanding social problems are linked either to an analysis of power or one of individual pathology. In many cases, the words used to describe a problem are coded ways of talking about race and racism. In addition, they reflect assumptions about other issues; issues about class, gender inequality, age and sexuality (Ridley 2005).

Therefore, a key starting point in the shifting of social work practice from a focus on individual pathology to one based on an analysis of power is to consider the terms that are used to describe social problems. In the current debates about social work and social activism, concepts such as diversity, empowerment and building self-esteem have come to signify a particular orientation to professional practice that is geared towards changing people rather than changing institutions. I call this a 'charity' approach to social work, and one that is based on a benevolent paternalistic sense of helping less fortunate people.

Deploying anti-racist strategies

Alternatively, an anti-racism strategy allows for a reconsideration of the underlying assumptions of power in society and the control of disadvantaged people of colour by discriminatory institutions (Solomos 2000). My argument here is not that race is the 'master narrative' that trumps all other forms of oppression. Rather, I am arguing that given the concentration of disadvantage that exists in communities of colour across the world, racism gives us a good lens and a starting point for understanding the need for a social justice approach to social work practice. Anti-racist interventions help to counter the tendency to take a 'charity' response to problems that originate from social inequality rather than individual pathology.

To be clear, social workers are very skilled at providing important social services. The profession has developed a wide array of methods to support people who have faced traumatic events. We have developed intervention programmes geared towards helping people develop new behavioural skills, we have elaborate therapeutic models that facilitate individual change, interpersonal relationships and group dynamics. All of these counselling, educational and self-help programmes are important ways to minimize pain and suffering. Income support programmes, therapeutic nurseries, mental health agencies, substance abuse treatment and prisoner re-entry programmes are all examples of essential direct services (Rubin 2000).

Social workers are also strong advocates, demanding that institutions respond in more favourable ways to people who need assistance. Advocacy is a key part of the repertoire of professional work because it reflects a commitment to facilitating access to the human services that people in crisis need. Advocacy is based on a recognition of a citizen's rights to state services and access to public resources (Noble 2004). Using my work as an example, advocacy includes working with hospitals to demand that rape victims are treated respectfully, working with legal services to be sure that they protect the rights of children in state care, and working with immigrant groups who are demanding services that are linguistically accessible. When acting as advocates, social workers use knowledge about institutions, professional privilege and a commitment to equal opportunity to demand that people get what they deserve from institutions.

The limitation of both direct services and advocacy work is that neither one addresses the root causes of social problems. Direct services, no matter how effective they are, respond to symptoms, and advocacy substitutes the voice of a social worker for the voices of the people: people are not gaining access to institutions because they themselves demand it, but because the social worker, by acting as an advocate, has ensured such access. Therefore, neither direct services nor advocacy work fully to address issues of power.

Instead, we need to consider approaches to social care that look at the root causes of problems. Concretely, this approach would allow social workers to consider what it would mean if we assumed radical political positions about injustice in addition to the very important work we do to help people heal. It would enable a focus on the part of social work that is about community organizing itself to change the conditions that disadvantage people, and it would require a shift in social workers' identity such that our own professional reputation would be less important than the extent to which we were accountable to our clients (Mizrahi 2001). It becomes important to determine which social workers are willing to risk the loss of professional power and prestige by assuming such a position. In addition, even if we can imagine such an approach to social work, there are limited models of practice that can help professionals realize more radical goals. However, such goals should include:

1 Reallocating resources to those who are most disadvantaged.
2 Building a community's capacity to care for itself instead of relying on professionals or outside institutions for help.
3 Disrupting institutional practices that actually *create* social inequality, including charity work.

In my view, working towards such goals requires attention to the various forms of oppression that people of colour and other disadvantaged groups face.

Anti-racist work against violence to women

I will draw upon my own experience as an activist social worker to illustrate the importance of anti-racist praxis. Violence against women is a very serious problem that affects all segments of the world's population (Weldon 2002). It has been declared a major health problem and an economic crisis, and is one of the most significant barriers to improving women's lives in both the developed and the developing world (Sudbury 2005). However, it is important to understand that the impact of violence against women is not felt equally among those women with privilege and those who are most disadvantaged. In the US context, it is the case that 25 per cent of all women experience intimate partner violence regardless of their socioeconomic status (Bureau of Justice Statistics 1995). However, there is clear evidence that women of colour, poor women, prostitutes, women with substance abuse problems and immigrant women are more likely to face the worst consequences of gender violence (Sokoloff 2005).

This fact requires social workers who work to prevent violence against women to include an analysis of racism as part of the experience of gender oppression. To do so, it is imperative that violence be defined broadly, beyond interpersonal violence and sexual assault from acquaintances and strangers to include racist state violence, the violence associated with poverty, racially motivated hate crime and the abuse associated with mean-spirited public policy and war (Richie forthcoming).

When violence against women is understood in this way, activist social workers will be compelled to avoid strategies that rely too heavily on the criminal legal system to solve the problem, because of the problematic experiences that women of colour and other members of our community have in the face of the criminal legal system. In addition, it means that organizations must pay particular attention to the consequences of accepting funding that places restrictions on services to immigrant women, lesbian women in abusive relationships or women with criminal backgrounds because of their addition to illegal substances. Furthermore, such an approach prohibits us from building coalitions with institutions that require that we base our work on a compromised, non-critical analysis of the ways that the state enforces racial domination.

Strategic steps towards anti-racist practice

The initial step in considering the development of an anti-racist strategy is for social workers to conduct a cultural self-assessment. This requires an in-depth and honest evaluation of one's values, attitudes, expectations and assumptions with regard to different ethnicities. The self-assessment should include a review of one's exposure to a rage of cultural practices and one's openness to considering alternative analyses of social problems.

The second step requires social workers to create an inventory of their access to culturally relevant information regarding the populations with which they are working. This would include not only published scholarly analyses of the historical and contemporary issues that a community faces, but also access to the patterns of everyday life and the various influences on behaviour that are unique to different communities. Social workers then need to develop a broad social and political analysis of the problems that individuals who live in disadvantaged circumstances face. This step requires that social workers broaden their understanding of individual problems by thinking about larger questions of inequality, discrimination, isolation and institutional racism as the root causes of many social problems. The next step is to consider how the current individual approach to social work practice is not only insufficient, but can potentially cause harm to certain social groups. The final step is to shift the intervention paradigm by adding social justice work to the direct services and advocacy approach. Here social workers will be required to work for social change through community development and by encouraging changes in public policy, as well as advancing social consciousness about racism and other forms of oppression. This step must include monitoring the work, being accountable to the populations being served and engaging in a constant iterative process with colleagues about the importance of anti-racist praxis as a fundamental aspect of social work intervention.

In conclusion, anti-racism intervention and activism in social work practice means more than doing outreach to bring more people of colour, more women, more queer people, more immigrant groups or more prisoners into our services. That would be merely 'colouring up' the same old way of doing things. Instead, it means being intentional about using strategies for organization against racial domination as well as personal change, and moving beyond individual charity work. It requires that we fundamentally change the nature of the work: the analysis of social problems needs to be more focused on root causes, intervention strategies need to more accurately reflect the full circumstances of the population in need, and we must build multicultural organizations where power is shared. The extent to which our work succeeds depends on how closely we link an analysis of social problems to the issue of oppression. Activist social workers and the organizations that they work in have a responsibility to make this link, working to liberate those people who 'present' in as being in need.

References

Bennett, L., Riger, S., Schewe, P., Howard, A. and Wasco, S. (2004) Effectiveness of hotline, advocacy counseling and shelter services for victims of domestic violence, *Journal of Interpersonal Violence*, 19(7): 815–29.

Bureau of Justice Statistics (1995) *National Crime Victimization Survey: Preventing Violence Against Women*. Washington, DC: National Institute of Justice.

Franklin, C. (2001) Coming to terms with the business of direct practice and social work, *Research on Social Work Practice*, 11(2): 235–44.

Gambrill, E. (2001) Social work: an authority-based profession, *Research on Social Work Practice*, 11(2): 166–75.

Goodkind, S. (2005) Gender-specific services in the juvenile justice system: a critical examination, *AFFILIA*, 20(1): 52–70.

Herivel, T. and Wright, P. (2003) *Prison Nation*. New York: Routledge.

Mizrahi, T. (2001) The satus of community organizing in 2000: community practice context, complexities, contradictions and contributions, *Research on Social Work Practice*, 11(2): 176–89.

Noble, C. (2004) Postmodern thinking: where is it taking social work? *Journal of Social Work*, 4(3): 289–304.

Ridley, C. (2005) *Overcoming Unintentional Racism in Counselling and Therapy: A Practioner's Guide to Intentional Intervention*. Thousand Oaks, CA: Sage.

Richie, B. (forthcoming) *Black Women, Male Violence and the Build-up of A Prison Nation*.

Rubin, A. (2000) Social work research at the turn of the millennium: progress and challenges, *Research on Social Work Practice*, 10: 9–14.

Sokoloff, N. (ed.) (2005) *Domestic Violence at the Margins: Readings on Race, Class, Gender and Culture*. New Brunswick, NJ: Rutgers University Press.

Solomos, J. (2000) *Theories of Race and Racism: A Reader.* New York: Routledge.

Sudbury, J. (ed.) (2005) *Global Lockdown: Race, Gender and The Prison-Industrial Complex.* New York: Routledge.

EXERCISE 1

Being clear about effective interventions

> The facilitator should ask students to consider the following quote from earlier in this chapter:

> > In my view, it is not good enough to keep developing more services – even if they are good services – and providing them in greater doses to those who are most disadvantaged in our society. In fact, a practice that merely offers services as people's troubles mount could, by some measures, be considered irresponsible.

> Students should then divide up into small groups of five to seven to consider this statement. Each group should sequentially respond to the following questions:

> 1. What do we mean by being disadvantaged?
> 2. What is an effective helper?
> 3. Where services are provided by an agency which are specifically 'contracted', for example providing welfare rights information, to what extent does this undermine wider issues relating to poverty, inequality and structural change?
> 4. In the participants' own work, can they identify experiences in their practice where they felt their intervention was 'short term' and relatively limited in effectiveness?

 EXERCISE 2

Exploring labels and individualizing problems

> Students should consider this quote from Beth's contribution:

> > Therefore, a key starting point in the shifting of social work practice from a focus on individual pathology to one based on an analysis of power is to consider the terms that are used to describe social problems. In the current debates about social work and social activism, concepts such as diversity, empowerment and building self-esteem have come

to signify a particular orientation to professional practice that is geared towards changing people rather than changing institutions.

The quote suggests that much of our work in the helping professions contextualizes problems in terms of 'the individual'. Students should be given a list of key words which denote particular categories of 'user':

- An asylum-seeker
- A depressed person
- An abused child
- An older person who is isolated and vulnerable
- A single parent Asian woman Living on a housing estate and suffering racist attacks
- A sex offender in community
- A young person involved in local crime and substance misuse
- A young person coerced to sell their body

How would the above individuals be given 'service provision' (if any) by an individual worker? Students should consider what the wider social causes are in relation to the above. For example, for 'A sex offender in the community', responses might include:

- Counselling relating to abuse caused to others
- An individual treatment programme
- Coordinating a multi-agency response to track the offender

A wider societal response may include:

- Developing ways of changing men's power
- Exploring community empowerment to become aware of potentially harmful men
- Wider national and international understanding and resourcing of a range of high profile campaigns of awareness of the issues surrounding sex offenders

 EXERCISE 3

Theorizing the context of intervention

The extent to which our work succeeds depends on how closely we link an analysis of social problems to the issue of *oppression.* Activist social workers and the organizations that they work in have a responsibility to make this link, working to *liberate* those people who 'present' in as being in need.

Students should be encouraged to consider the following key words, define them and discuss them in relation to their practice:

- Oppression
- Liberation

Students should:

- Research the origins of these two words
- Consider when they first appeared in the literature of their profession
- Explore what each word means in terms of their day-to-day work
- Be asked to undertake some project work in which the participants identify an area of social work and social care that requires a radical form of intervention; for example, where existing forms of intervention and/or assessment are structured in such a way that they do not take into account wider societal influences. Participants should then report back their finding and present the evidence for their conclusions.

Students who are embarking on their first year of qualification may want to think about how they could work collaboratively with university staff and communities to develop an effective resource. This does not have to be a massive undertaking, but could be a small area, street, or community which has structural problems and needs acivism and focus. This would require diplomacy and planning, and the community members should always be central to all that is explored.

chapter **five**

SOCIAL WORK AND SOCIAL VALUE: WELL-BEING, CHOICE AND PUBLIC SERVICE REFORM

Bill Jordan

Values are not private, spiritual or metaphysical beliefs. They are – or should be – the standards by which we judge actions and justify our decisions. But how are values related to *value* – the worth attached to people, animals and material resources?

Human well-being depends on access to goods that confer value. In affluent, commercial societies, material goods are accessible mainly through markets and government agencies. How then do people convert material goods into self-esteem and subjective well-being (overall satisfaction with quality of life)? And which interpersonal goods matter most to people?

Until recently, economists – as the dominant social science profession and the main influence on government – dismissed these questions as meaningless. They argued that, because preferences for goods vary between individuals, we must allow each (as far as possible) to choose their own ingredients for a good life, within an infrastructure of rules for fairness among citizens. Now, leading theorists such as Layard (2005) suggest that there is evidence from psychological research (Kahneman *et al.* 1999; Huppert *et al.* 2005) to indicate clearly what makes people happy with themselves and their lives (Helliwell 2003). Although in any society, better-off people enjoy more subjective well-being (SWB) on average than poor ones, some countries with relatively low incomes per head have higher levels of SWB than would be predicted, and the SWB levels of populations in affluent states have failed to rise with growing incomes in the past 40 or 50 years (Frey and Stutzer 2002).

The factors that contribute most to SWB are health, job satisfaction and relationships – close personal ties, friendships and involvement in the community (Helliwell 2003). So it is psychological, relational and interpersonal (social) elements which most contribute to well-being. This implies that all value, including the economic value that is signalled by prices, salaries and property portfolios, must be understood within a framework of *social value*. I shall argue that social work is a profession which deals in social value, but that this has been systematically obscured by recent government policies and organizational reforms (Jordan 2007b).

Economists' belated interest in well-being signifies that they are catching up with other social scientists and human service professionals. The distinguished anthropologist, Mary Douglas (1978: 190), pointed out that all human interactions take place within cultures that provide 'the cost-structure and distribution of advantages which are the contexts of everyday decisions, as well as the legacy of past exchanges'. In order to gain value of any kind, one has to subject oneself to the cultural standards which apply to one's actions. Service users explain their situations and their needs in these terms, and social workers respond as much as members of the same moral and political community as they do as experts or bureaucratic assessors.

So social value is produced and exchanged through interactions within cultures for the evaluation of character, behaviour and quality. Social work is, by its own professional claims, primarily concerned with improving well-being through relationships, both with and between service users (see e.g. Shulman 1999: 22, 35; Adams *et al.* 2005: 2). It seeks agreed criteria for what is good and right, and tries to help people in various kinds of need and trouble attain these standards. As in all other interactions, social work may produce stigma, blame, guilt, exclusion and shame; however, it tries to minimize these losses of social value.

Cultures and social institutions provide the means for translating experience (including the consumption of material goods) into social value, and hence well-being. The economic historian, Avner Offer (2006), has shown that individualism, commercial innovation and the instant gratifications of consumer spending have weakened cultural ways of transforming raw experience into quality in a context of interpersonal exchanges of 'regard'. This applies to restraining, pacing and sequencing such activities as eating, drinking, shopping, moving around, dating, socializing and raising children. It helps to explain the rise of obesity, binge drinking, addiction, debt and family breakdown in the UK and USA. In addressing such issues, social work is trying to help people revalue themselves and each other, and develop practices of emotional closeness, respect and participation, against the tide of commercialization and instant gratification.

In all the anglophone countries, economic restructuring and public sector reform have been associated with increased stress and unhappiness (Lane 2000; Pusey 2003). Social work tries to help people produce and exchange more social value through their everyday interactions (Garfinkel 1967; Goffman 1969), while commercial advertising and government rhetoric tell them that they are primarily rational economic agents, seeking 'independence', 'positional advantage' and 'self-realization' (Hirsch 1977; Jordan 1996). The logic of consumer choice sees each individual as a utility-maximizer in an order based on contracts. Such a culture of competition, unconstrained by social boundaries, in which groups are provisional and temporary and status negotiable, leaves individuals and contracts as the only 'sacred' sources of value (Douglas 1978: 192). Government policy points people away from social support, loyalty and the secure sense of belonging, and towards short-term material satisfactions and instrumental strategies for advantage over others.

Independence and interdependence

Thus social work values must seek to bridge social and economic versions of value to reconcile two fundamentally different perspectives on human society. The one which prevailed at the birth of western modernity was that it was (or should be) a voluntary association between free individuals, who agreed the rules under which they lived together. In the theories of Locke, Montesquieu, Hume and Rousseau, equal individual freedom was the basis of all other political and social institutions; but this freedom relied on rights in property – self-ownership, which forbade tyranny, and exclusive ownership of material resources (Macpherson 1962). All previous systems of relationships (such as feudalism and theocracy) were declared unethical and contrary to natural rights, but commercial exchange under capitalism was pronounced the economic counterpart to government by consent (Hirschman 1977).

From an alternative, feminist, perspective Carole Pateman (1988, 1989) has pointed out that this new order incorporated women as 'natural subordinates', because they were seen as too emotional and unruly for reliable self-government. At the same time, it relegated the household, the informal economy and such unorganized relationships as friendship and community to a secondary position or substratum of the 'real' business of the economy and politics. As an activity initiated by middle-class women for remoralizing their working-class fellows, and focusing mainly on the household and informal community life, social work accepted this status in its formative years.

It is interesting to see how social work's codes of ethics and values struggle to deal with this differentiation of status between the dominant rights of liberal democracy (inherited from the Enlightenment), and the subordinate priorities of the family and communal relations (see Chapter 2). Individual freedom and dignity occupy a prime position, followed by social justice – the distributive role of government – and a commitment to professional probity and competence. Even anti-oppressive values have been assimilated into this framework, which defines value in terms of individual self-ownership and rationality.

However, some feminist writers have argued for a radical challenge to the priorities of modern liberal capitalism. Following from Elshtain's (1981) advocacy of 'maternal' values and practices, writers such as Tronto (1993), Williams (2001) and Meagher and Parton (2001) have suggested that an 'ethic of care' would be a better basis, both for society and for professional practice. So far, this has not been adequately reflected in professional ethics.

The essential difference between the two approaches is that, instead of upholding the 'independence' of the individual over unwarranted infringements of liberty, the feminist perspective starts from the inescapable interdependence of social relations, and considers how the benefits of this can be maximized. In the economic model which now supplies the theory of public service reform, interdependence occurs when individuals can impose costs on each other (such as crime, pollution or crowding), or when private rights cannot be assigned (Buchanan and Tullock 1962). Government exists to deal with 'external effects' and to maximize individual choice; it is about the *unavoidable* interdependence that stems from sharing a limited number of material resources and public amenities.

During New Labour's administrations, as under the Conservatives since 1979, policy and management in the UK have moved towards enabling citizens to control their own access to services, previously seen as a sphere of equal and shared democratic participation. Nowhere are these goals clearer than in the government's 'vision for adult social care', entitled *Independence, Wellbeing and Choice* (DoH 2005), which sees individual budgets for the purchase of care as the ideal for this sector.

If social workers are really to uphold the value of emotional support, empathy, mutuality, respect and belonging (the positive products of social interactions), then this is a partial and incomplete account of social care. Being able to buy from alternative suppliers is only truly beneficial if their staff genuinely value those who need help, and give them the chance to contribute to social value (for instance, in groups and communities), as well as receive practical assistance. Conversely, those who give such care should be more highly valued and rewarded. The report of the Parliamentary Committee on Human Rights has shown that these standards are far from being realized (BBC Radio 4 2007).

Even more strikingly, the finding that the UK was 21st out of 25 European Union (EU) member states in the league table for the well-being of children and young people (Bradshaw *et al.* 2007) was followed by the revelation that it was bottom of 21 affluent Organization for Economic Cooperation and Development

(OECD) states, just below the USA (Innocenti Report 2007). Despite good outcomes for educational attainment, the UK's children scored particularly badly for self-assessed well-being, peer and family relationships, and for risky behaviour. The top performers, predictably, were the Scandinavian countries and the Netherlands, but the Mediterranean countries (Spain, Italy, Slovenia, Malta, Cyprus and Greece) all did much better than the UK. This suggests that valuing children and giving them self-esteem does not only depend on a specific set of public services (generously funded in the Scandinavian countries) or pattern of family life (the latter have many working mothers and single-parent households), but also on a coherence and mutual consistency between the institutions sustaining childhood. In the Mediterranean countries, family, church, kinship and neighbourhood reinforce each other (Jordan 2006a).

The well-being perspective can therefore provide very different insights into quality of life from the ones which derive from the economic model, if social value, friendship and community become more significant than consumption opportunities, autonomy or choice. This is more in line with the goals and methods of social work: but the assertion of the established list of professional values has done little to ensure that the well-being perspective is needed.

Social value and the service economy

A good way to look at the differences between an approach which takes social value into account and present UK government strategies is the rationale for the expansion of the service sector. Most private expenditure, and around 70 per cent of employment, is now in services. This sector includes banking, finance and insurance, the UK's most significant roles in the global economy, and the activities which generate most of our income from abroad. However, most service employment is now in the public services, or in private sector retailing, social care, hospitality, recreation and cleaning – low paid, personal services, subsidized by tax credits and enforced by benefit authorities (Jordan with Jordan 2000; Jordan 2006b).

The government's rationale for the continued growth of the latter kinds of commercial services is that they provide the jobs which enable people to escape from poverty and dependence on benefits. This justifies extending the requirement to be actively seeking work, first to people claiming invalidity benefit who are judged to be capable of some paid employment, and then to lone parents with children at secondary school. The implication is that work of this kind will go on expanding, as more and more activities which used to be informal are commercialized. People (mainly women) who previously cooked, gardened and cared for themselves, and looked after their own children and parents, will go out to work, and do the same things for other (better-off) people, who earn much more, or can afford not to be employed.

The government's claims about routes out of poverty look thin against the findings that the UK has the lowest rates of social mobility among the affluent OECD nations (Sutton Trust 2007), and the highest rates of inequality since the mid-1980s (Joseph Rowntree Foundation 2007). It is clear that, as in the USA, a service economy which creates employment of a menial kind increases money incomes, but at the expense of consolidating differentials of opportunity, wealth and power. The kinds of work that are created are often demeaning and exploitative (Abrams 2002; Ehrenreich 2002).

Within this model, any kind of paid work, however routine or mechanical, servile or demanding, is better than unpaid activity, even if the latter is creative, affirming and socially valuable in terms of the self-esteem and enhancement of well-being it achieves. Conversely, any kind of paid service is worth more to those who receive it than doing things for oneself, or doing them informally with others. Because the economy grows as paid services expand, this is by definition welfare-improving.

I have argued that the evidence of the failure of children's and adults' SWB to rise in line with incomes is a damning indictment of this approach. Instead of using the power of state officials to impose service work on poor people, and the tax-benefit system to subsidize low-wage, menial services for the better-off, our society needs to find new ways to make the value we get from our relationships with each other – as partners, parents, friends and members of communities – recognizable, and to promote this rather than commercial service employment. There ought to be a level playing field on which unpaid social roles and communal activities can compete with paid ones, and people can indicate which they value most, rather than being steered or bullied into commercial exchanges (Jordan 2007a). Interdependence, not individual independence, should be enabled.

The irony of social policy, for example, in the UK during the past ten years, has been that the New Labour government has genuinely tried to address the neglect of deprived individuals and districts that occurred under Conservative administrations. Its policies for social inclusion, urban regeneration, community cohesion, respect and now well-being have all attempted to engage with disaffected individuals and groups, so as to improve social relations where they have been most anomic, conflictual or deviant (Jordan with Jordan 2000; Jordan 2006c). But all this has been more than offset by the emphasis on individual autonomy, property and self-realization as the bases for the mainstream order. Because the better-off have been enabled to seek advantage in the educational, health and welfare systems, this has more than cancelled out the gains achieved by New Labour's initiatives on inclusion and community.

As Douglas (1978) has argued, individualism, competition, contract and the cult of celebrity are all parts of a culture which makes the other forms of interpersonal value – stemming from emotion, affection, respect, loyalty and belonging – invisible, or actively devalues them. Unless social work can form alliances in a movement against this culture, its practice will tend to reflect these same values, or be constrained by them.

Conclusions

Well-being research and theory directs attention from quantity of material consumption to quality of experience. In this way, it favours the approach to value taken by social work, especially in its concern with relationships. Now that economists are paying attention to qualitative elements in happiness (Ainslie 1992, 2001), to empathy and emotional communication (Sugden 2005), and to interpersonal exchanges of 'regard' (Offer 2006), there is an opportunity for social work to reassert its historic priorities in more confident ways.

If a serious attempt is made to evaluate the quality of work in social care, and with children in need, this will redirect attention back to the value which people get and give through face-to-face interactions. It will reverse the 20-year trend towards seeing social work as a technical, competence-based activity, 'delivering' individualized bits of service to meet practical needs, or packages of intervention to change people's behaviour.

The shift which is needed to achieve this can be compared with the one required for environmental sustainability. Just as we are waking up to the need to value natural resources, biodiversity, habitats and wild places to avoid ecological catastrophe, so too will we have to value each other – as friends, neighbours and fellow citizens – more explicitly and through our actions, if we are to increase well-being. Like all culture shifts, this calls for changes in the organizational contexts of our lives, in our images and the ideas by which we steer our behaviour, and not just in our beliefs and rhetoric.

References

Abrams, F. (2002) *Below the Breadline: Life on the Minimum Wage*. London: Profile Books.

Adams, R., Dominelli, L. and Payne, M. (eds) (2005) *Social Work Futures: Crossing Boundaries, Transforming Practice*. Basingstoke: Palgrave.

Ainslie, G. (1992) *Picoeconomics: The Interaction of Successive Motivational States Within the Person*. Cambridge: Cambridge University Press.

Ainslie, G. (2001) *Breakdown of Will*. Cambridge: Cambridge University Press.

BBC Radio 4 (2007) *News*, 15 August.

Bradshaw, J. Hoelscher, P. and Richardson, D. (2007) An index of child well-being in the European Union 25, *Journal of Social Indicators Research*, 80: 133–79.

Buchanan, J.M. and Tullock, G. (1962) *The Calculus of Consent: Logical Foundations of Constitutional Democracy*. Ann Arbor, MI: Univeristy of Michigan Press.

DoH (Department of Health) (2005) *Independence, Well-being and Choice: Our Vision for the Future of Social Care for Adults in England*. London: DoH.

Douglas, M. (1978) Cultural bias, in *In the Active Voice*. London: Routledge & Kegan Paul.

Ehrenreich, B. (2002) *Nickel and Dimed: Undercover in Low-Wage America*. London: Granta Books.

Elshstain, J.B. (1981) *Public Man, Private Woman: Women in Social and Political Thought*. Oxford: Martin Robertson.

Frey, B. and Stutzer, A. (2002) *Happiness and Economics: How the Economy and Institutions Influence Well-being*. Princeton, NJ: Princeton University Press.

Garfinkel, H. (1967) *Studies in Ethnomethodology*. Englewood Cliffs, NJ: Prentice Hall.

Goffman, E. (1969) *Interaction Ritual*. Harmondsworth: Penguin.

Helliwell, J.F. (2003) How's life? Combining individual and national variables to explain subjective well-being, *Economic Modelling*, 20: 331–60.

Hirsch, F. (1977) *Social Limits of Growth*. London: Routledge & Kegan Paul.

Hirschman, A.O. (1977) *The Passions and the Interests: Arguments for Capitalism Before its Triumph*. Cambridge, MA: Harvard University Press.

Huppert, F.A., Baylis, N. and Keverne, B. (2005) *The Science of Well-being*. Oxford: Oxford University Press.

Innocenti Report (2007) *Child Poverty in Perspective: An Overview of Child Well-being in Rich Countries*. Florence: UNICEF.

Jordan, B. (1996) *A Theory of Poverty and Social Exclusion*. Cambridge: Polity.

Jordan, B. (2006a) Well-being: the next revolution in children's services?, *Journal of Children's Services*, 1: 41–50.

Jordan, B. (2006b) Public services and the service economy: individualism and the choice agenda, *Journal of Social Policy*, 30(1): 143–62.

Jordan, B. (2006c) *Social Policy for the Twenty-First Century: New Perspectives, Big Issues*. Cambridge: Polity.

Jordan, B. (2007a) *A Theory of Poverty and Social Exclusion*, 2nd edn. Cambridge: Polity.

Jordan, B. (2007b) *Social Work and Well-being*. Lyme Regis: Russell House.

Jordan, B. with Jordan, C. (2000) *Social Work and the Third Way: Tough Love as Social Policy*. London: Sage.

Joseph Rowntree Foundation (2007) *Inequality in the United Kingdom*. York: Joseph Rowntree Foundation.

Kahneman, D., Diener, E. and Schwartz, N. (eds) (1999) *Well-being: The Foundations of Hedonic Psychology*. New York: Russell Sage Foundation.

Lane, R.E. (2000) *The Loss of Happiness in Market Democracies*. New Haven, CT: Yale University Press.

Layard, R. (2005) *Happiness: Lessons from a New Science*. London: Allen Lane.

Macpherson, C.B. (1962) *The Political Theory of Possessive Individualism: Hobbes to Locke*. Oxford: Oxford University Press.

Meagher, G. and Parton, N. (2001) Modernising social work and the ethics of care, *Social Work and Society*, 2(1): 10–26.

Offer, A. (2006) *The Challenge of Affluence: Self-Control and Well-being in Britain and the United States Since 1950*. Oxford: Oxford University Press.

Pateman, C. (1988) *The Sexual Contract*. Cambridge: Polity.

Pateman, C. (1989) *The Disorder of Women: Democracy, Feminism and Political Theory*. Cambridge: Polity.

Pusey, M. (2003) *The Experience of Middle Australia: The Dark Side of Economic Reforms*. Cambridge: Cambridge University Press.

Shulman, L. (1999) *The Skills of Helping Individuals, Families, Groups and Communities*, 4th edn. Ithaca, NY: Peacock.

Sugden, R. (2005) Correspondence of sentiments: an explanation of pleasure in social interaction, in L. Bruni and P.L. Porta (eds) *Economics and Happiness: Framing the Analysis*, pp. 147–62. Oxford: Oxford University Press.

Sutton Trust (2007) *Social Mobility in Britain*. London: Sutton Trust.

Williams, F. (2001) In and beyond New Labour: towards a new political ethics of care, *Critical Social Policy*, 21(4): 467–93.

EXERCISE 1

Define your 'leisure' time

> This exercise requests that we consider what we 'do' with time we have which is not work-related. The facilitator should encourage students to work in small groups and list the range of activities they engage in. The list may be extensive. When it is completed it should be compiled by a facilitator and then, systematically, students should go through each activity and assess which is paid for and which has no cost attached. For example, visiting family is not necessarily 'cost related' but to get there may cost money in terms of transport, purchasing flowers and so on, hence the primary activity is free, but there could be a cost and consumption elements involved.
>
> The exercise is attempting to find out the subtlety of consumer activity. This can be made into a game where groups attempt to catch each other out in terms of what activities they choose to do and whether there are 'purchases' (hidden or otherwise) or not.

  EXERCISE 2

What do you value?

> The challenge of Bill Jordan's chapter is that it asks us to reassess the priorities of what are the central activities of society. In a society based on 'consumption' we can all become engrossed in activities which, according to Jordan's argument, do not benefit us (our health and well-being) in the long term. In this exercise students 'monitor' their activities and experience of 'our world' in terms of what is promoted in society – what do they do with their leisure time? Does this require them to 'purchase things' or focus on other activities? How much depends on their parting with money?
>
> Students need to be made conscious of how we are often, without realizing it, 'captive' to every purchase, however small, and they should keep a daily log, listing their experience of this throughout the course of a week. This is, in some ways, a strange exercise where students' activities are reflected on in terms of their very existence!

Students should report back and share their findings in small groups.

 EXERCISE 3

Workers as an agents provocateur?

Students should consider the following quote from Bill Jordan's chapter:

> *social work is trying to help people revalue themselves and each other, and develop practices of emotional closeness, respect and participation, against the tide of commercialization and instant gratification.*

1 How do social workers/care workers do this?
2 Should they do this?
3 Does it contradict how we ourselves live our lives?
4 Do you agree with the overall thrust of Bill Jordan's chapter?

There are no easy answers to these questions, but they should provoke a very lively debate.

 EXERCISE 4

The quest for 'well being': an unhappy society?

In Bill Jordan's chapter one of his central themes is how we define 'well-being' and how we achieve it. This exercise encourages students to explore the extent of 'contentment' and 'unhappiness' in our society. Some field work is required, and students can undertake the work individually or in groups.

1 How do we measure contentment in our own country – is there a way of measuring it?
2 Is the rate of diagnosed illnesses (related to unhappiness) going up or down? For example, depression may be a 'classification' we could explore, or more extreme, suicide.
3 Is there a 'plan' nationally or locally to help combat increasing problems with mental health?

4   Who are the most contented people in the country – is there
    a measure? Some countries have criteria for this; try to find
    out the measures used.

chapter six

SERVICE USER VALUES FOR SOCIAL WORK AND SOCIAL CARE

Peter Beresford

Social work has historically prioritized values of autonomy and self-determination for service users, and these continue to be central in the formal statements about its purpose produced by its institutions and organizations. Thus, social work's international bodies describe its objectives as to promote:

> social change, problem solving in human relationships, and the empowerment and liberation of people to enhance well-being. Utilising theories of human behaviour and social systems, social work intervenes at the point where people interact with their environments. Principles of human rights and social justice are fundamental to social work.
>
> (IFSW 2001)

The General Social Care Council (GSCC), which is responsible for the regulation of social work and social care in England, has developed a code of practice for social care workers. This states that workers must:

- protect the rights and promote the interests of service users and carers;
- establish and maintain the trust and confidence of service users and carers;
- promote the independence of service users while protecting them as far as possible from any danger of harm;
- respect the rights of service users while seeking to ensure that their behaviour does not harm themselves or other people;
- uphold public trust and confidence in social care services;
- be accountable for the quality of work and take responsibility for maintaining and improving knowledge and skills (see www.gscc.org.uk).

However, there is no one uniform approach to social work. It ranges from the radical social work developed in the 1970s (Langan and Lee 1989) and the social justice-based models advanced by writers like Holman (1993), Jordan (1990) and Jones (Jones and Novak 1999), to the care management which has become a dominant strand of contemporary social work practice, institutionalized in statutory services for adults. Few analysts would agree that the latter serves the liberatory purposes with which social work has sought to associate itself (e.g. Postle 2001, 2002). Furthermore, other more judgemental values are often not far from the surface of social work. Thus, for example, in a modern and much reprinted standard social work textbook, we can read the following summation of social work's challenges:

> What can we offer people who show 'neurotic tendencies'; who cannot give 'good-enough' parenting; who seem to be insatiably dependent on others; who block out their emotions; and who 'act out' rather than talk through their difficulties, albeit that these are usually underlying rather than presenting problems.
>
> (Coulshed and Orme 1998: 133)

The problem of excluding service users

Until recently, the development and discussion of social work values has tended to be typified by one enduring characteristic. The focus of these values, the voluntary or involuntary recipients of its services – traditionally called 'clients', now more often known as 'service users' – have had little or no say in the debate. Their views have not been sought. Their role in the construction of social work, in so far as they have had one, has been as a data source to be harvested, rather than as a stakeholder to be engaged.

The suggestion here is that this is an essentially paternalistic approach to developing the value and knowledge base of the profession and discipline, especially given its own privileging of people's autonomy and self-determination. There seems to be a fundamental contradiction between such values and social work's own model of development. Now that there are professional and political requirements that service users and their perspectives be fully involved in social work, this tradition clearly needs to be challenged. It is also difficult to see how, without including service users and their views, ideas and experiences, it is likely to be possible to achieve either a workable value base for social work or one which has any lasting or agreed legitimacy.

The importance of service users' perspectives

Increasing interest in service users' views means that these are now finding their way into professional literature as well as service users' own writings. However, it is important to remember that service user discussions have historically largely been hidden, informal and oral in tradition. While service users are critical of poor-quality social workers, they have many positive things to say about those they see as supportive and helpful. Service users stress that they want workers who truly listen to them, who treat them with equality and respect, who value and understand diversity, who show empathy and warmth towards them, are reliable, well informed and understand the barriers that face them, and work with them to challenge such barriers. They consistently talk about the key human qualities they value in social workers as well as their skills. Good social workers are clearly seen to be people with particular personal qualities as well as professional skills.

Service users also value and refer to the underpinning *social* approach of good social workers, preferring it to the essentially medicalized approach of many other professionals they encounter. This is significant. Ultimately, what makes social work *social* work is that it is inherently concerned – in theory at least – with the *social* as well as (but not instead of) the personal. A tension in much social work has been that often it is only seen to have the capacity to intervene in the personal, rather than the social. Nonetheless, this consciousness of both aspects of people's lives – the personal and the social – and their complex interactions and interrelations, along with the desire to understand and acknowledge both, lies at the heart of formal conceptions of social work and has been one of its great strengths. This is of importance to many service users. Much of the philosophical and theoretical developments pioneered by service users and their movements (most conspicuously that of disabled people) has prioritized social approaches and seen them as key to moving from oppressive and discriminatory structures, understandings and ways of working, to anti-discriminatory and more egalitarian ones (Oliver 1996; Oliver and Barnes 1998).

Counter-pressures at work

However, social work's value base has to be considered in the context of the wider sociopolitical environment in which it operates – one which, in more recent years particularly, has often been harsh and unsympathetic to social work. Statutory social work continues to be under-resourced, overloaded, low valued and susceptible to other people's ideas and agendas. A White Paper, *Our Health, Our Care, Our Say*, published in 2006, had little to say about the role of social workers (DoH 2006). Social work, like other public services, has also been heavily influenced by the dominance of managerialist approaches which have had far-reaching effects. Thus, heavy external pressures have been at work on the organization and development of social work, particularly state social work, which have tended to pull it away from its own stated value base.

Meanwhile, a series of values and concepts have been emphasized by government and become both the context of social work and the directions in which it is supposed (rhetorically at least) to be going. It is these values which I want to focus on in this discussion, because not only have they become central to government ideology, they are also concepts and values which are identified and highlighted by service users and their movements. These key concepts and values are: choice; partnership; social inclusion; empowerment; user involvement; citizenship; and independence. There may be others to address too, but these seem to be some of the most important. All are key concerns in current discussions, rhetoric and public policy relating to social work and social care. All are equally to be found at the heart of service user discussions and literature.

Exploring competing values and understandings

I want to consider some of the contests and struggles that are going on around these ideas and values. I aim to consider their meanings from two points of view – that of government and of service users – because this is likely to help us clarify our own understanding and goals, both in relation to social work values generally, and specifically in relation to service user values for social work.

Choice

The UK government, like its recent predecessors, is emphatic about the central importance of *choice* in public services for the public, for patients and for service users. The rhetoric is now strongly established that there needs to be 'consumer choice' in public provision. We should be able to choose the service we use and the professional who provides it. The government has framed the choice agenda in terms of having options of service, and the key route it has developed to achieve this is a shift to the market – to the private sector and private financing. This was originally presented as part of a 'third way' in politics, based on a new mix of state and market (Giddens 1998).

Service users also highlight choice and opportunity, but report that they often receive poor-quality services from *all* sectors: public, private and voluntary. In social care, all the evidence highlights that the one case where people feel they have gained more choice has been direct payments – fully accessible and properly operated – where they are in control of their support. It is *being in control*, not merely having different service providers, which continue to provide the same old services, that they stress they want (Beresford *et al.* 2005; Branfield *et al.* 2005).

Partnership

Government also calls for 'partnership'. There are increasing requirements to show evidence of partnership with citizens', community and service users' organizations in local planning, commissioning and providing arrangements. Service users want partnerships too, to work in close association with service planners and providers, in order to ensure that problems are anticipated before they emerge. But service users ask, how do you make partnership work (Shaping Our Lives 2007)? How do you make it real when individual service users may be overloaded with their own difficulties, service user organizations are generally insecure and underfunded, and practitioners frequently do not feel adequately supported by their organizations (Branfield *et al.* 2005)? What value do such partnerships have in the context of the business imperatives now operating with contracting and private finance initiatives? Service users stress the importance of having their own adequately and securely funded service-user controlled organizations to make such partnerships meaningful. Such a network was advocated in 2005 by the Prime Minister's Strategy Unit, but at present service users' organizations seem to be being run down rather than strengthened (Branfield *et al.* 2006).

Social inclusion

When 'New Labour' came to power in 1997, it placed a new stress in the UK on the idea of 'social inclusion' as one of its core public policy concepts. It expressed a strong commitment to challenging 'social exclusion'. But social *inclusion* has since increasingly been officially associated with inclusion in the labour market – that is to say, being in paid employment (Levitas 2005). This has been reflected in an increasing pressure for service users to move 'from welfare to work', an emphasis on people fulfilling 'social obligations' as a prior basis for receipt of social entitlements; government rhetoric of 'work for those who can, security for those who can't'; and reform of the benefits system. A strong tension has emerged between integration and assimilation.

Many service users wish to contribute through working, but also want to do so through education and training, and through getting involved in their communities. Many feel under pressure to move into employment – any employment – regardless of its quality, their capacity to maintain it, or its responsiveness to their particular needs and difficulties. Meanwhile, service users, particularly mental health service users, report pressure to come off benefits. For them, social inclusion tends to mean something very different: challenging the discrimination and stigma which marginalize them, safeguarding their rights, ensuring their participation in public and social institutions, and supporting personal and social relationships.

Empowerment

The idea of empowerment grew out of the black civil rights movement in the USA and has been an inspiration to many movements since, including service user movements. It has now come to be used by governments, policy-makers and the market often to mean encouraging both service users and workforces to take more responsibility. Its definition has become vague in the process. It has also tended to be diluted to mean 'feeling good', with a narrow focus on personal empowerment – a focus on changing yourself and how you feel about yourself (Baistow 1995; Croft and Beresford 1995).

Service users tend to reject professional definitions of empowerment, which are based on requiring conformity with the prescriptions of services and service workers. For them empowerment has indivisible personal and political aspects. It means being able to make change in ourselves to raise our self-esteem, expectations and abilities, so that we can bring about broader social and political change. That is why, despite the damage done by the overusage of the term, it continues to be valued by service users and their organizations. Crucially, it unifies the personal and the political, highlights the need to address both, and supports service users to challenge their powerlessness (Croft and Beresford 1995; Shera and Wells 1999).

User involvement

User involvement is perhaps the concept and value that has been most open to competing interpretations. Crucially, government and the public service system have borrowed language and ideas from the market to define user involvement in terms of drawing people in to offer their views and experience to inform what the state and services should ideally do. This approach has resulted in a kind of state market research, sometimes on a giant scale, like the consultation meeting held in Birmingham and attended by some 1000 people which was used to inform the production of the 2006 primary health and social care white paper (DoH 2006). This model of participation or user involvement is perhaps best described as 'managerialist/consumerist'. The balance and distribution of power essentially remain unchanged. Service users' views serve as a data source to inform policy-makers and the locus of decision-making in the policy-making process remains the same.

For service users, user involvement typically means having a say and being able to influence services that impact upon them and the lives they lead. Their approach to involvement is best understood as a 'democratic' one, where the aim is to change the balance of power and to influence decision-making, both within organizations and services and in people's own lives. If direct payments offer people individual control, then the purpose of such user involvement is to offer service users collective influence and control over policy and provision (Beresford and Croft 1993; Barnes and Mercer 2006). No wonder there is so much talk of tokenism and tick-box exercises when service user democratic aspirations for involvement come into collision with consumerist approaches to delivering it.

Citizenship

Issues and values relating to citizenship have been central in New Labour government policies and thinking. Sadly, however, for a government wedded to positive ideas like stakeholding, social inclusion and involvement, it feels as if the emphasis has been on the negatives, rather than the positives. The focus has not been on what we can expect as citizens – not on rights, entitlements and indeed, responsibilities. Instead it has been on who should *not* be a citizen; who should be denied the rights and responsibilities of citizenship and on restricting further the health and welfare entitlements of those included in this category as refugees and asylum seekers (Cohen 2005). An emphasis on the denial of citizenship rights, closely associated with the populist agenda of the right-wing press, has become the defining issue of UK citizenship discussion. Social work and social care have been sucked into this as part of the apparatus of policing this system (Humphries and Hayes 2004).

Meanwhile, service users have placed a very different emphasis on citizenship. They have made it one of the defining ideas of their value system. Service users, starting with the disabled people's movement and gradually extending to other user groups, have placed a crucial emphasis on a *rights*-based approach to their lives and to the social care services which are intended to support them. Instead of talking about 'needs' and 'needs-based' services, which has historically tended to result in one group defining the needs of another, service users have sought to underpin health, social care and welfare with a civil and human rights model which is geared to taking account of and securing their rights (Campbell and Oliver 1996; Beresford and Campbell 2004).

Independence

Both government and the main opposition parties have frequently stressed the significance of 'independence', particularly in relation to welfare policy. The term has mainly been used to mean encouraging self-reliance, 'standing on your own two feet' and managing without help. Independence has been presented as a virtuous value and contrasted with dependence on welfare benefits, failure to maintain social obligations, social breakdown and the existence of a disaffiliated 'underclass'. It has served to stigmatize several groups, notably lone parents, mental health service users and people who are long-term unemployed.

Independence has emerged as a value of at least as much importance to service users. It has gained particular prominence because of its association with the idea of 'independent living' pioneered by the international disabled people's movement. This followed from their development of the social model of disability. This model is a further expression of a rights-based approach, since it highlights the need to challenge the barriers which restrict people's lives, choices and opportunities. The idea of 'independent living' turns on their head traditional ideas of expecting service users to manage unaided, redefining it instead to highlight the need for people to have the support they require to live their lives independently on as equal terms as possible with other people (Morris 1993; Oliver 1996; Swain *et al.* 2004).

Conclusion

These seven values and ideas set the political context of contemporary social work and social care. They are at the heart of their own value base and central to service users. All are strongly contested, with widely different meanings attached to them. The question is: which of these competing meanings will prevail in social work and social care? Will it be the significantly regressive meanings adopted by government, or the progressive versions of these values which service users and their movements have developed? While the language is the same, these interpretations point in very different directions.

Social work and social care have long had a struggle over whether their primary function is a controlling or liberatory one. Perhaps they will always have dual responsibilities where, to secure the rights of some, they must restrict the rights of others. But this is not the same as primarily being an agent of social control. Unless social work and social care sign up to the liberatory values of service users, it is difficult to see how current goals of putting service users at their heart will be achieved. Instead, they are likely to be tied to an inherently controlling role that will leave them marginalized and unable ever to command public support and regard.

This leads to a final question. How is a democratic, rights-based and emancipatory approach to social work and social care, based on service user values, to be achieved? Over the last 15 to 20 years, the structures of social work and social care have been increasingly shaped by outside political, ideological and managerial interests. Social work identifies itself as a profession, yet since the community care reforms, the independence and discretion of social workers have been more and more constrained as they have been subjected to budget-driven decision-making. Politicians, policy-makers, senior managers and local authority bureaucrats have been the key shapers of modern social work. With weak professional organizations and limited collective organization, face-to-face practitioners have only a minor role in the leadership or decision-making of social work and social care.

What is needed now are new alliances, particularly between service users and face-to-face practitioners (Beresford and Croft

2004). There are many overlaps between the two. The social care workforce faces many forms of marginalization. It includes high proportions of women and members of black and minority ethnic communities, many of whom are living on low incomes. The same is true for service users. There are many overlaps between service workers and users to build on, as well as differences. By linking and working together behind the progressive values advanced by service users, there is a real chance for social care and social work to become the truly liberatory systems of support that they have the potential to be.

References

Baistow, K. (1995) Liberation and regulation: some paradoxes of empowerment, *Critical Social Policy*, 14(3): 34–46.

Barnes, C. and Mercer, G. (2006) *Independent Futures: Creating User-led Disability Services in a Disabling Society*. Bristol: Policy Press.

Beresford, P. and Campbell, P. (2004) Participation and protest: mental health service users/survivors, in M.J. Todd and G. Taylor (eds) *Democracy and Participation: Popular Protest and New Social Movements*. London: Merlin Press.

Beresford, P. and Croft, S. (1993) *Citizen Involvement: A Practical Guide for Change*. Basingstoke: Macmillan.

Beresford, P. and Croft, S. (2004) Service users and practitioners reunited: the key component for social work reform, special issue, *The Future of Social Work*, *British Journal of Social Work*, 34 (January): 53–68.

Beresford, P., Shamash, O., Forrest, V., Turner, M. and Branfield, F. (2005) *Developing Social Care: Service Users' Vision for Adult Support* (report of a consultation on the future of adult social care), *Adult Services Report 07*. London: Social Care Institute for Excellence in association with Shaping Our Lives.

Branfield, F., Beresford, P., Danagher, N. and Webb, R. (2005) *Independence, Wellbeing and Choice: A Response to the Green Paper on Adult Social Care* (report of a consultation with service users). London: National Centre for Independent Living and Shaping Our Lives.

Branfield, F. and Beresford, P. with Andrews, E.J., Chambers, P., Staddon, P., Wise, G. and Williams-Findlay, B. (2006) *Making User Involvement Work: Supporting Service use Networking and Knowledge*. York: Joseph Rowntree Foundation.

Campbell, J. and Oliver, M. (1996) *Disability Politics: Understanding our Past, Changing our Future*. London: Routledge.

Cohen, S. (2005) *Deportation is Freedom: The Orwellian World of Immigration Controls*. London: Jessica Kingsley.

Coulshed, V. and Orme, J. (1998) *Social Work Practice: An Introduction*. Basingstoke: Macmillan.

Croft, S. and Beresford, P. (1995) Whose empowerment? Equalising the competing discourses in community care, in R. Jacks (ed.) *Empowerment In Community Care*. London: Chapman & Hall.

DoH (Department of Health) (2006) *Our Health, Our Care, Our Say: A New Direction for Community Services*. London: The Stationery Office.

Giddens, A. (1998) *The Third Way: The Renewal of Social Democracy*. Cambridge: Polity Press.

Holman, B. (1993), *A New Deal for Social Welfare*. Oxford: Lion Publishing.

Humphries, B. and Hayes, D. (eds) (2004) *Social Work, Immigration and Asylum: Debates, Dilemmas and Ethical Issues for Social Work*. London: Jessica Kingsley.

IFSW (International Federation of Social Workers) (2001) Definition of social work, www.ifsw.org/en/p38000208.html, accessed 6 June 2007.

Jones, C. and Novak, T. (1999) *Poverty, Welfare and the Disciplinary State*. London: Routledge.

Jordan, B. (1990) *Social Work in an Unjust Society*. London: Harvester Wheatsheaf.

Langan, M. and Lee, P. (eds) (1989) *Radical Social Work Today: Social Work in the Recession*. London: Hutchinson.

Levitas, R. (2005) *Inclusive Society? Social Exclusion and New Labour*. Basingstoke: Palgrave Macmillan.

Morris, J. (1993) *Independent Lives: Community Care and Disabled People*. Basingstoke: Macmillan.

Oliver, M. (1996) *The Politics Of Disablement*. Basingstoke: Macmillan.

Oliver, M. and Barnes, C. (1998) *Disabled People and Social Policy: From Exclusion to Inclusion*. London: Longman.

Postle, K. (2001) 'The social work side is disappearing. I guess it started with us being called care managers', *Practice* 13(1): 13–26.

Postle, K. (2002) Working 'between the idea and the reality': ambiguities and tensions in care managers' work, *British Journal of Social Work*, 32: 335–51.

Prime Minister's Strategy Unit (2005) *Improving the Life Chances of Disabled People*. London: The Stationery Office.

Shaping Our Lives (2007) Partnership working: service users and social workers learning and working together, in M. Lymbery and K. Postle (eds) *Social Work: A Companion to Learning*. London: Sage.

Shera, W. and Wells, L.M. (eds) (1999) *Empowerment Practice in Social Work: Developing Richer Conceptual Foundations*. Toronto: Canadian Scholars' Press Inc.

Swain, J., French, S., Barnes, C. and Thomas, C. (eds) 2004) *Disabling Barriers: Enabling Environments*, 2nd edn. London: Sage.

EXERCISE 1

What do you call people you work with?

> This is a quick and simple exercise. Students should think about and discuss what terms they feel most comfortable in using in relation to those they work with. Apart from exploring people's ideas about preferred language, this is also a 'trick' exercise in that it makes an 'assumption' that it is the worker who needs to be made 'comfortable' with what they call 'users' and that *they* make that decision. An extension of this is to then think of scenarios where workers 'patronize' users – i.e. addressing them as 'love' or 'dear'.

 EXERCISE 2

Empathy with being a service user

> Students should get into twos and threes and then think in turn of a time when they did not feel heard by a service or organization to the point where they could have or should have complained. When the exercise is done in twos and threes students can join larger groups up and share their experiences in a wider group. The facilitator then asks each student to report back and a nominated person will need to highlight key points and link common themes/experiences.

 EXERCISE 3

Ingredients that go towards being 'user empowered'

> This exercise requires students to undertake some work in advance. Students should divide into small groups and allocate the following areas to be explored:
>
> 1   The history of 'user informed/led' services.
> 2   Models of working with users.
> 3   Examples of 'best practice' when working with users.
> 4   Examples of poor practice when working with users.

5   Organizations which promote good practice when working with users.
6   Key theorists in the subject.

 EXERCISE 4

How much do users (students) shape the education they get?

> How much 'say' do students have in the 'etching' and development of the education they get? Do they have a great deal of say – where in the curriculum is their 'handprint'? What proportion of what is taught can honestly be said to be shaped by students *and* the service users they work with? How could this be improved?
>
> Students should consult the 'Shaping Our Lives' website on models of good practice – see www.shapingourlives.org.uk.

 EXERCISE 5

Thinking about the disempowered

> Students need to think about the most disempowered groups in society – those who have their liberty taken from them, those forced into doing things they find hard (e.g. young people who are failing at school). The question is: how, using the theories and values underpinned in this chapter, could they be helped to shape the service they receive?

chapter **seven**

COMMUNITY INTERVENTION AND SOCIAL ACTIVISM

Vishanthie Sewpaul

This chapter deals with the ideological underpinnings of the concept of 'community', with the term generally being imbued with positive connotations of collective solidarity and 'being for the other' as exemplified in the philosophy of *uBuntu* in the South African context. The chapter argues that the values typically ascribed to communities have become appropriated by right-wing conservatives and in the name of principles such as 'self-reliance', 'moral regeneration' and 'partnerships', governments are increasingly shifting the burdens of care onto local communities. In the face of this, the chapter argues that community interventions based on social activism, advocacy and lobbying are key strategies in the process of 'organizing from below' in order to keep governments accountable to their people and to enhance the quality of life for local communities.

Conceptualizing community

The concept of 'community' is variously conceived (e.g. Leonard 1997; Dominelli 2004), with the following two views gaining primacy in social work literature. A community may be conceived of as groups of people who, although diverse, live in and share a specific geographic space within common mezzo-level infrastructural development. Community has also been defined in relation to a group of people that share a common interest, where people may be spatially separate and indeed may never physically meet. For example, the mission statement of the International Association of Schools of Social Work (IASSW) makes reference to 'a community of social work educators', implying that despite huge diversities, social work educators around the world might be bound by some common threads and that that they might be able to coalesce around some common agendas.[1] The Treatment Action Campaign (TAC) in South Africa is another example. The TAC consists of an association of people at local and national levels, who have successfully networked with like-minded non-governmental organizations (NGOs) on an international level to exert pressure on the South African government and on the multinational drug companies to make anti-retroviral treatment accessible. Leonard (1997: 155) speaks of *imagined communities* as social movements 'which consist of those who *apply* for the rights and responsibilities of belonging, whose subject positions include a certain commitment to a set of ideas, even though some of them may be internally contested'. Such communities, Leonard argues, have 'a strength which is lacking in that other kind of community in which membership is automatic or taken for granted, a community of proximity and common culture as a way of life, where the subject experiences effortless belonging' (p. 155).

However one conceives of 'community', the concept is generally imbued with positive connotations of: a common solidarity; people coming together to work toward some common goals; altruism, sharing and benevolence; and social and economic interdependence. Although critical of Tonnies's (1952) conception of *Gemeinshaft* as 'communities as unifying forces' (Dominelli 2004: 203), with the argument that such a conception contributes to suppression of diversities and to the dynamics of inclusion and exclusion, Dominelli concludes that (p. 204):

> Communities provide spaces in which people seek and gain approval, are reaffirmed in their interests or sense of who they are and what they stand for, participate in key decisions, and negotiate with others around issues of change and stability ... Dignity, reciprocity, interdependence and solidarity provide the ties that bind communities and disparate people together.

Borrowing on Tonnies's typology of *Gemeinshaft* and *Gesellschaft*, Pawar and Cox (2004: 10) differentiate between traditional and modern communities, with the former characterized by a locality base, common culture, sense of identity and sense of belonging, and the latter geographically dispersed, multicultural and providing a partial sense of identity where 'belongingness' depends on common interests. Traditional communities should not be idealized or rarefied; negative attributes also abound. Pawar (2004) posits that humanistic postmodernism with its focus on human orientation, reflexivity and sensitivity for the aesthetic, the particular and the excluded, has the potential to constrain or eradicate the 'mean spirited, superstitious, religious, constraining, authoritarian and backward' (Pawar 2004: 256) characteristics of traditional community, while also having the potential to counter the negative aspects of modernism in relation to alienation, individualism, increased consumerism, greed and environmental degradation.

Ubuntu: an African conceptualization of community

Under apartheid, the majority of South Africa's people (almost 80 per cent of the population that were not classified white) suffered the most atrocious forms of human degradation. Black Africans were relegated to the very bottom of the social strata and were subject to extreme poverty and deprivation in all areas of life, while people of all hues who opposed apartheid were subject to detention without trial, and ran the risk of torture and death.[2] Post-apartheid South Africa saw the reclamation of African values and norms, with efforts to inscribe *Ubuntu* as part of our national consciousness and as part of nation-building. The philosophy of *Ubuntu* is reflected in the African adage (isiZulu language) *'umuntu ngumuntu ngabantu'*, that is, 'a person is a person through other persons'. *Ubuntu* emphasizes the equality and dignity of all human beings, the sanctity of life, collective solidarity that enhances group care and self-reliance, compassion and respect. It is a philosophy that was invoked by people like Nelson Mandela and Archbishop Desmond Tutu in South Africa's path to peace and reconciliation post-1994 and perhaps, in no small measure, contributed to South Africa's exemplary transition from apartheid to peaceful democracy. Given our history, revenge, a desire for the annihilation of the oppressor, anarchy and war could have been the alternatives that fortunately gave way to that of *Ubuntu*.

However, like the limitations of traditional communities, *Ubuntu* does have its drawbacks. The emphasis on group solidarity, consensus and community could degenerate into a 'total communalism' (Sono 1994: xiii) where individuals who advance beyond the community are marginalized and where the group, as so eloquently articulated by Sono (1994: 7), could be:

> overwhelming, totalistic, even totalitarian. Group psychology, though parochially and narrowly based ... nonetheless pretends universality. This mentality, this psychology is stronger on belief than on reason; on sameness than on difference. Discursive rationality is overwhelmed by emotional identity, by the obsession to identify with and by the longing to conform to. To agree is more important than to disagree; conformity is cherished more than innovation. Tradition is venerated, continuity revered, change feared and difference shunned. Heresies [i.e. the innovative creations of intellectual African individuals, or refusal to participate in communalism] are not tolerated in such communities.

Neo-liberal capitalist appropriation of *Ubuntu*

Important in the South African context is that *Ubuntu's* emphasis on community and group care has been exploited by the state to abdicate its responsibility to people. The vision of the *White Paper for Social Welfare* reads: 'A welfare system which facilitates the development of human capacity and self-reliance within a caring and enabling socio-economic environment' (Department of Welfare and Population Development 1997). It is unfortunate that subsequent welfare policies seem to have latched on to the development of self-reliance, rather than focusing on the creation of a caring and an enabling socioeconomic environment to facilitate self-reliance. The *Draft National Family Policy* (hereafter referred to as 'the *Policy*') (Department of Social Development 2005), produced in January 2005, is filled with ideological inconsistencies reminiscent of an apartheid, albeit a non-racialized, ideology, as detailed by Sewpaul (2005). The *Policy* is underscored by South Africa's neo-liberal economic policy – *Growth, Employment and Redistribution* (GEAR) (Ministry of Finance 1996).[3]

It begins with the following situational analysis (p. 5), adopting a conservative, morally judgemental and residual approach to family and community living:

> In the second decade of democracy, South Africans continue to suffer the ravages of an oppressive and exploitative legacy. The long-term effects of apartheid, migrant labour, land displacement, rapid urbanisation, and poor rural development, amongst others, may require no less than a generation to redress. Add to this widespread poverty, escalating incidences of HIV infection and AIDS, rampant domestic violence and rape, growing sexual abuse of children, and increasing crime and drug trafficking, and hope for the future becomes even bleaker.

The above is immediately followed by: 'In all of this *the family remains the crux* of how South Africans cope – or fail to cope – in a society challenged with *rebuilding the moral fibre within individuals and amongst communities*' (p. 6, emphasis added). There are two obvious problems with such an approach. Firstly, the burden of coping with South Africa's huge problems is reduced to the level of individuals, families and local communities, without recognition of the structural sources of unemployment, economic oppression and exclusion, inequality and poverty on people's lives and the profound roles that society and state play in contributing to how people cope. Secondly, 'rebuilding the moral fibre within individuals and amongst communities' appears to be the panacea for all of the problems mentioned. The document also makes ten additional calls for the moral regeneration of communities (see Sewpaul 2005 for details). The subtext suggests that morally corrupt families and communities lead to morally corrupt societies. Therefore, the corollary argument asserts that *rebuilding the moral fibre within individuals and communities* will ensure the *restoration of the moral fibre of society.*

The language contained in the text presumes the existence of external resources for families. Sewpaul (2005) asserts that the *Policy* pathologizes families, with its focus on the development of inner resilience, self-reliance and capacitating families without creating dependence. While the *Policy* constantly speaks of the need for 'self-reliance' (a term often used to abdicate state responsibility towards the people), the Human Sciences Research Council's report (Amoateng *et al.* 2004) boldly asserts that the majority of families in South Africa are currently not self-reliant on account of external constraints. As social workers, we need to ask: if external socioeconomic, political and cultural factors are maintaining communities in poor, dispossessed and helpless positions, how are such communities expected to move toward independence and self-reliance within the same structural constraints?

Responsibility, freedom and development

Liberal democracy, exemplified by neo-liberal capitalism, in the guise of expanding individual freedom and choice, and facilitating self-reliance and responsibility, all too often constrains choices in terms of access to health, education, welfare and information (Amin 2001; Sewpaul 2006). We need to adopt a dialogical and interactive approach towards the relationship between freedom, responsibility and development, as advocated by Sen (1999), who addresses the intrinsic and instrumental values of freedom. Sen argues that while individual agency and freedom are central to addressing all forms of social, economic and political deprivation, 'the freedom of agency that we individually have is inescapably qualified and constrained by the social, political and economic opportunities that are available to us' (pp. xi–ii). Sen contends that the removal of substantial 'unfreedoms', such as lack of freedom to access food, shelter, health and education and to participate freely in the labour market (the alternative to such participation might be bonded or slave labour) is constitutive of development. Yet, Sen (2005: 201) places a high premium on the value of freedom to think and on the importance of argument, dialogue and debate – on democratic participation:

' ... the weakness of voices of protest has helped to make the progress of social opportunities unnecessarily slow'. Sen (1999: 284) maintains that:

> Responsibility *requires* freedom. The argument for social support in expanding people's freedom can, therefore, be seen as an argument *for* individual responsibility, not against it ... Without the substantial freedom and capability to do something, a person cannot be responsible for doing it ... freedom and capability to do something does impose on the person the duty to consider whether to do it or not, and this does involve individual responsibility ... freedom is both necessary and sufficient for responsibility.

In saying this, Sen is contesting the view of right-wing conservatives that provision of public services creates dependency and detracts from individual responsibility, and the view that self-reliance and responsibility might be antithetical to each other. Simply put, for example, parental responsibility to care for their children depends on socioeconomic conditions that allow for those responsibilities to be fulfilled. The value of Sen's contribution is that he does not present freedom as the absence of restraint: the call is for positive freedoms that enhance human capabilities and responsible living (Hall and Midgley 2004).

One of the lobby campaigns in South Africa is for a basic income grant (BIG), where the lobbyists might be constructed as a 'community of interest' across spatial divides. South Africans should come together in a collective solidarity to support the BIG coalition and the call of the Minister of Social Development, Dr Zola Skiweyi, for a BIG. It is extremely disappointing that the state president, Thabo Mbeki, and the Minister of Finance, both dismiss the possibility of a BIG. The refusal to consider a BIG is often premised on the all too common, albeit misguided, assumption that it will either cause or reinforce dependency and laziness, and contribute to a deepening moral decay of society, as people will misuse the unearned money. The assumption is also that a 'meagre' amount of R100 per month per person will make little or no difference, reflecting a lack of understanding of the survival strategies adopted by poor people. Poor people living in extreme poverty generally live in larger households. If a poor household has, for example, 10 unemployed members, there might be no income whatsoever at the end of each month. Should each person in that household receive R100 per month, this would result in an income of R1000 per month (about US$140). Certainly no offer of luxury, but potentially the difference between life and death. Contrary to popular opinion that a BIG would lead to dependence and laziness, research produced by the Economic Policy Research Institute (EPRI 2001, 2002) and Samson *et al.* (2004) indicates that households that receive social security are better able to seek and obtain employment. There is a simple logic to this. With no income at all, people have no funds to make telephone calls or pay for public transport to get to a job interview. The EPRI revealed that the partial means-tested grants close the poverty gap by 23 per cent but nevertheless exclude those poorest households that do not have members receiving unemployment benefit, state pensions, disability grants or include children qualifying for grants. Even with full uptake of the existing grants, for those who qualify within the designated categories, such grants would reduce the poverty gap by only 36 per cent. With universal coverage, a BIG (most of which could be recovered through a system of progressive taxation and thus constitute a non-threatening means of redistribution) would close the poverty gap by about 74 per cent (EPRI 2001).

Social security promotes job search and employment opportunities, increases school attendance, decreases expenditure on healthcare, reduces hunger and nutritional deficiencies (all of which are important social development indicators – Samson *et al.* 2004) and provides some measure of economic freedom for people to exercise some choice and responsibility. Increased access to education produces other benefits. For example, the Word Bank (cited in Samson *et al.* 2004) found a positive link between education and preventing the spread of HIV/AIDS. The authors (p. 134) concluded that empirical evidence demonstrates that:

> People in households receiving social grants have increased both their labour force participation and employment rates faster than those who live in households that do not receive social grants. In addition, workers in households receiving social grants have realized more rapid wage increases. These findings are consistent with the hypothesis that South Africa's social grants increase both the supply and demand for labour. This evidence does not support the hypothesis that South Africa's system of social grants negatively affects employment creation.

It is unfortunate that, despite strong calls from the Minister of Social Development and concerned citizens, and empirical evidence indicating the potential developmental benefits of a BIG, the South African government refuses to consider it, and advocates instead principles of individual and community self-reliance, partnerships and responsibility, as manifested in its emphasis on income generation projects and contract-based public work programmes. Discourses in the public sector in South Africa have often equated community development with income generation, entrepreneurship and micro-credit lending schemes (Dominelli 2004). Dominelli argues that an emphasis on self-help and people's own capacities to overcome disadvantage has 'depoliticized community work and drawn it into the ambit of techno-bureaucrats and competence-based appraisal schemes. Its crucial weakness is relating to residents as excluded people without engaging in the necessary structural changes, particularly the polarization of wealth' (2004: 207).

Community intervention and social activism in South Africa

While conventional community intervention strategies in the form of community organization, community education and awareness around specific issues such as teenage pregnancy, HIV/AIDS and disability, income generation and developing entrepreneurship remain dominant among social workers and community development practitioners, a new social movement, based on the mobilization of communities from below is gaining ground in South Africa.[4] This has been most marked in the Landless People's Movement, in people's struggle to access water, electricity and housing, and in people's efforts to work towards alternative forms of globalization (Desai 2002; Hart 2002; Bond 2004, 2005; Naidoo and Veriava 2005). Desai (2002), writing nine years after the first democratic elections in South Africa that spelled hope and a better life for millions of people, describes people's disillusionment with the African National Congress, and how local communities have formed social forums and coalitions to challenge the brutality of municipalities in their struggle against water and electricity cut-offs and evictions from their homes. Desai asserts that 'Rivulets of humanity were back on the streets demanding land, a basic income grant, anti-AIDS medication, a halt to privatization, and dignity' (p. 11).

Within the framework of neo-liberal capitalism, which involves the promotion of corporate interests, and those of the International Monetary Fund, the World Bank and the World Trade Organization (WTO), it is the survival and rights of the poor, of workers and of women that are grossly compromised (Klein 2000; Fortunato Jr 2005; Lebowitz 2005; Magdoff and

Magdoff 2005). The growing inequalities engendered by global capitalism, the denial to millions of people of access to basic services such as food, water, shelter and gainful employment, and the relegation of millions of people to disease, death and poverty have all been well documented (Hoogvelt 1997; Amin 2001; Desai 2002; Hart 2002; Terreblanche 2002; Bond 2004, 2005; Magdoff and Magdoff 2005; Saul 2006; Sewpaul 2006). There are undoubtedly huge discrepancies between the quality of life of those in the developed north and those in the global south, the following being just a few examples. McNally (2002) cites the WTO which claims that, on average, an American earned 5500 per cent more than an Ethiopian. According to Magdoff and Magdoff (2005), the wealthiest 691 people in the world have a net worth of US$2.2 trillion, equivalent to the combined gross domestic product (GDP) of 145 countries – more than all of Latin America and Africa combined. The richest 7.7 million people (about 0.1 per cent of the world's population) control approximately US$28.8 trillion – equivalent to 80 per cent of the annual GDP of all the countries of the world.

If social workers and community development practitioners are to make a contribution to the ending of poverty and inequality (Sachs 2005), we have no option but to engage in advocacy, lobbying and social activism at different levels. The relative absence of these in mainstream social work and state-funded and state-subsidized community development practice in South Africa has generated criticism from radical civil society organizations engaged in social activism. Sachs (2005), Desai (2002), Bond (2004, 2005), Brecher *et al.* (2002) and Naidoo and Veriava (2005) highlight the power of social movements in generating change at local, national and global levels, with Sachs arguing that the peaceful non-violent activism of Gandhi, the civil rights movement of Martin Luther King, and the revolts against the slave trade were all successful not because they made economic sense but because they had moral and ethical appeal. In a similar vein, pressure needs to be put on nation states, on the rich countries, especially the USA, and on the global financial institutions to work toward a fairer and more just world. Such an approach constitutes more than a moral appeal. It is pragmatic; it is in the common interest of all of humanity. Oppression, poverty and inequality are breeding grounds for resistance, which sometimes takes violent form, and can translate into 'terrorism'.

In order to be advocates and lobbyists, and in order to mobilize local communities in their struggle against hunger, illness, denial of education, healthcare and clean drinking water, we need to educate ourselves about the dynamics of power at local, national, regional and global levels. We need to understand how skewed development gets reproduced in the interests of the elite and how race, class and gender intersect with other social factors to deny some groups of people (primarily black people and especially black women) access to status, power, privilege and resources (Dominelli 2002, 2004; Sewpaul 2003, 2006). Given the hegemonic discourses around liberal democracy, and its concomitant neo-liberal capitalism (Mullaly 1993; Amin 2001; Sewpaul 2003, 2006; Bond 2005; Neocosmos 2005), many of us have difficulty thinking outside the system. Citing Marcuse, Mullaly (1993: 159) argues that:

> this hegemonic ruling process is so successful that most people cannot even conceive of any alternative to capitalism ... the ruling class alliance has managed to secure through the state such a total social authority over the subordinate classes that it shapes the whole direction of social life in its own interests.

Envisioning an alternative world order means that we put radical theory in moral terms: we need to understand that 'market forces are not driven by nature but are rather the results of human actions that generate conditions profoundly offensive to every extant religious and ethical system' (Fortunato Jr 2005: 9). Raising our own consciousness and the consciousness of the communities with which we engage is vital to our envisioning another world order or, in the words of Sachs (2005: 358), an 'enlightened globalization' that sees the end of poverty by 2025. Transforming 'common sense' into 'good sense' (Gramsci 1971)[5] is central to such as endeavour. The mechanism for such transformation lies in communities developing reflexive knowledge of the constraining forces of dominant ideologies and practices. Leonard (1997: 142) argues that 'given the massive legitimating power of dominant ideology in late capitalism, the project of emancipation might be seen as securing freedom from *self-imposed* constraints ... to distinguish the truth of the oppressed from the ideology of the oppressors'.

Based on community and social action strategies, Ferguson and Lafayette (2006) call for a social work of resistance, while Leonard (1997: 139–40) calls for 'organised collective political resistance ... [to confront] the cultural and economic monolith of the global market'. Adopting a postmodern approach to welfare, Leonard exhorts us to 'extend the actual experience and realization of interdependence beyond the boundaries of a politics of identities, "imagined communities" or single issue community movements"' (p. 159). Citing Fischer and Kling, Leonard (p. 159) asserts the following, which is an apt conclusion to this chapter:

> Single community based efforts are not large enough to challenge the enormous power of corporate capital or centralized government. Because community problems almost always originate beyond local borders, the ability to effect change depends to a great extent upon building coalitions, alliances, networks and progressive political parties. The success of such efforts, however, ultimately will be based upon whether specific ways can be found to break down racial and cultural barriers that are so prevalent and threatening ... throughout the world.

Notes

1   Tangible manifestations can be seen in the IASSW's and IFSW's (International Federation of Social Workers) development of global standards for social work education and training (see Sewpaul and Jones 2005), the international definition of social work and the *International Code of Ethics*, and IFSW's and IASSW's efforts to take on advocacy functions at a global level.
2   For an excellent and very readable exposition of life in South Africa during apartheid see Rian Malan's *My Traitor's Heart* (1991). The depth and detail regarding the dehumanization that occurred during apartheid provided by Malan in part helps us to contextualize contemporary South African society, particularly in relation to violent crime. There seems little doubt that South African history, combined with high levels of poverty, unemployment and inequality, is contributing to high levels of crime and violence, despite the obvious success of the truth and reconcilliation process.
3   GEAR, rooted in a neo-liberal ideology with its emphasis on fiscal austerity, cutbacks in state expenditure, curbing of interest rates, privatization of state assets and basic services, casualization of labour and lowering of trade tariffs (Hart 2002; Bond 2004, 2005; Sewpaul and Hölscher 2004; Naidoo and Veriava 2005), detracts from a structural and social justice approach to community and family living. The very premises of GEAR are based on individualism, corporate competitive-

ness and profit-making that do not augur well for a country with a professed commitment to social justice and a developmental welfare approach (Sewpaul 2005). Contrary to the expectations of a post-apartheid state, we have exacerbated the inequality of the past, increased unemployment, widened the poverty gap, and are in the unenviable position of having about the highest rate of HIV/AIDS in the world (Desai 2002; Terreblanche 2002; Bond 2004, 2005).

4 These conventional strategies are important and laudable and may have a profound impact at the micro- and mezzo-levels of development. However, the limitations are that they generally pose no threat to dominant power structures; they do not call for a reordering of external sociopolitical, cultural and economic systems that maintain people in vulnerable, poor and excluded positions; and they generally do not include emancipatory educational strategies such as consciousness-raising and praxis, which are central to a deepening democracy (see Sewpaul 2003, which draws on the emancipatory pedagogies of Paulo Friere, Henry Giroux and Antonio Gramsci). By maintaining the system-stabilizing functions of community work and not engaging in power relations and structural change, we might effectively be part of the problem rather than the solution.

5 Central to the work of Gramsci is what he called *common sense* (also *contradictory consciousness*) and *good sense*. He contended that common sense functions without the benefit of critical interrogation. Common sense consists of the incoherent set of generally held assumptions and beliefs common to any given society, while good sense means practical, empirical common sense – thus the need to transform common sense into good sense.

References

Amin, S. (2001) Imperialism and globalization, *Monthly Review*, 53: 2, www.monthyreview.org/0601amin.htm.

Amoateng, A.Y. *et al.* (2004) *Describing the Structure and Needs of Families in South Africa: Towards the Development of a National Policy Framework for Families*. Pretoria: Child, Youth and Family Development Directorate, HSRC.

Bond, P. (2004) *Talk Left, Walk Right: South Africa's Frustrated Global Reforms*. Scottsville: University of KwaZulu Natal Press.

Bond, P. (2005) *Elite Transition: From Apartheid to Neoliberalism in South Africa*. Scottsville: University of KwaZulu Natal Press.

Brecher, J., Costello, T. and Smith, B. (2002) *Globalization from Below: The Power of Solidarity.* Cambridge: South End Press.

Department of Social Development (2005) *Draft National Family Policy* (January). Pretoria: Department of Social Development.

Department of Welfare and Population Development (1997) *White Paper for Social Welfare*, www.gov.za/whitepaper/1977. Pretoria: Department of Welfare and Population Development.

Desai, A. (2002) *We are the Poors: Community Struggles in Post-apartheid South Africa.* New York: Monthly Review Press.

Dominelli, L. (2002) *Anti-oppressive Social Work, Theory and Practice.* Basingstoke: Palgrave Macmillan.

Dominelli, L. (2004) *Social Work: Theory and Practice for a Changing Profession.* Cambridge: Polity Press.

EPRI (Economic Policy Research Institute) (2001) www.epri.org.za.

EPRI (Economic Policy Research Institute) (2002) www.epri.org.za.

Ferguson, I. and Lafayette, M. (2006). Globalisation and global justice: towards a social work of resistance, *International Social Work*, 49(3): 309–18.

Fortunato Jr, S.J. (2005) The soul of socialism: connecting with the people's values, *Monthly Review*, 57: 3, www.monthlyreview.org/0705fortunato.htm.

Gramsci, A. (1971) *Selections from the Prison Notebooks*, eds and trans A. Hoare and G.N. Smith. London: Lawrence & Wishart.

Hall, A. and Midgley, J. (2004) *Social Policy for Development.* London: Sage.

Hart, G. (2002) *Disabling Globalisation: Places of Power in Post-apartheid South Africa.* Pietermaritzburg: University of Natal Press.

Hoogvelt, A. (1997) *Globalization and the Postcolonial World: The New Political Economy of Development.* London: Macmillan.

Klein, N. (2000) *No Logo.* London: HarperCollins.

Lebowitz, M.A. (2005) The knowledge of a better world, *Monthly Review*, July-August, 57: 3, www.monthlyreview.org/0705lebowitz.htm.

Leonard, P. (1997) *Postmodern Welfare: Reconstructing an Emancipatory Project.* London: Sage.

Magdoff, H. and Magdoff, F. (2005) Approaching socialism, *Monthly Review*, 57: 3, www.monthlyreview.org/0705magdoffs1.htm.

Malan, R. (1991) *My Traitor's Heart.* London: Vintage.

McNally, D. (2002) *Another World is Possible: Globalization and Anti-capitalism.* Winnipeg: Arbeiter Ring.

Ministry of Finance (1996) *Growth, Employment and Redistribution: A Macroeconomic Strategy.* Pretoria: Ministry of Finance, www.gov.za/reports/1996.

Mullaly, R. (2003) *Structural Social Work.* Totonto: McClelland & Stewart Inc.

Naidoo, P. and Veriava, A. (2005) Re-membering movements: trade unions and new social movements in neoliberal South Africa, in *From Local Processes to Global Forces*, Centre for Civil Society Research Reports, vol. 1, University of KwaZulu Natal.

Neocosmos, M. (2005) Re-thinking politics today: elements of a critique of political liberalism in Southern Africa, in *From Local Processes to Global Forces,* Centre for Civil Society Research Reports, vol. 1, University of KwaZulu Natal.

Pawar, M. and Cox, D. (2004) *Community Informal Care and Welfare Systems: A Training Manual.* Centre for Rural Social Research, Charles Sturt University, New South Wales.

Sachs, J. (2005) *The End of Poverty: How Can We Make it Happen in Our Lifetime?* London: Penguin.

Samson, M. *et al.* (2004) *The Social and Economic Impact of South Africa's Social Security System,* final report. Claremont: Economic Policy Research Institute.

Saul, J.S. (2006) *Development after Globalization: Theory and Practice for the Embattled South in a New Age Imperialism.* London: Zed Books.

Sen, A. (1999) *Development as Freedom.* Oxford: Oxford University Press.

Sen, A. (2005) *The Argumentative Indian: Writings on Indian Culture, History and Identity.* London: Penguin.

Sewpaul, V. (2003) Reframing epistemologies and practice through international exchanges: global and local discourses in the development of critical consciousness, in L.D. Dominelli and W.T. Bernard (eds) *Broadening Horizons: International Exchanges in Social Work.* Aldershot: Ashgate.

Sewpaul, V. (2005) A structural social justice approach to family policy: a critique of the draft South African Family Policy, *Social Work/ Maatskaplike Werk,* 41(4): 310–22.

Scwpaul, V. (2006) The global-local dialectic: challenges for African scholarship and social work in a post-colonial world, *British Journal of Social Work,* 36: 419–34.

Sewpaul, V. and Hölscher, D. (2004) *Social Work in Times of Neoliberalism: A Postmodern Discourse.* Pretoria: Van Schaik Publishers.

Sewpaul, V. and Jones, D. (2005) Global standards for the education and training of the social work profession, *International Journal of Social Welfare,* 14(3): 218–30.

Sono, T. (1994) *Dilemmas of African intellectuals in South Africa.* Pretoria: UNISA.

Terreblanche, S. (2002) *A History of Inequality in South Africa 1652–2002.* Pietermaritzburg: University of Natal Press.

Tonnies, F. (1952) *Community and Association: Gemeinshaft und Gesellschaft.* London: RKP.

EXERCISE 1

Social workers as educators and community workers?

> Is there a 'common goal' in social work/community work as stated in this quote?

> > the mission statement of the International Association of Schools of Social Work (IASSW) makes reference to 'a community of social work educators', implying that despite huge diversities, social work educators around the world might be bound by some common threads and that they might be able to coalesce around some common agendas.

> Students should undertake some self-directed study exploring to what extent this is true for social work today in relation to communities. The following themes should be explored and then presented to the whole group:

> 1 What do we mean by 'a community of social work educators'? Can social workers be 'educators'?
> 2 Are social workers well placed to explore with communities what they can do to transform their lives?
> 3 Who are the primary 'thinkers' in relation to this issue?
> 4 When does social work become justified in helping others 'understand' what influences and shapes their lives and when is this notion 'political' manipulation?

  EXERCISE 2

Mapping your community

> The facilitator should provide each student with a large sheet of paper (flipchart size) and ask them to locate their own home in the centre of the sheet. They should then draw a local map of the streets nearby. Each student should identify who they know in those streets, what skills they have and whether these skills are used in the local community. The following questions should be addressed:

> 1 What skills exist in your local community?

2 Who is the oldest person in your local community?
3 Who has lived in the local community the longest?
4 Who is the most recent person to move into your local community?
5 Is there anyone with 'special needs' in your community?
6 Are there any 'skill-sharing' schemes in your local community?
7 Is there anyone who coordinates any activities in your local community?
8 How would you describe your local community?
9 What would you 'ideally' like to see your local community become?
10 Can you 'narrate' the type of community you live in?

This exercise often reveals that many communities exist in isolation. Students should be encouraged to think about how this situation might be changed.

 EXERCISE 3

Inequalities and community development

Students should be invited to consider the following quote:

> The richest 7.7 million people (about 0.1 per cent of the world's population) control approximately US$28.8 trillion – equivalent to 80 per cent of the annual GDP of all the countries of the world. If social workers and community development practitioners are to make a contribution to the ending of poverty and inequality (Sachs 2005), we have no option but to engage in advocacy, lobbying and social activism at different levels.

1 When you read this quote what comes to mind?
2 Do you deny this statistic or acknowledge it to be true?
3 Do you think it is the job of social work to be concerned or active in any way to alter this statistic?
4 What do you think you could do?
5 What would be the possible implications of your actions/commitments?
6 At what 'level' do you see your involvement?

chapter **eight**

ANTI-OPPRESSIVE PRACTICE AS CONTESTED PRACTICE

Lena Dominelli

Anti-oppressive practice (AOP) is a contested concept rooted in the values of equality and social justice. These values are underpinned by a belief in human rights and active citizenship – i.e., a state of belonging whereby people make decisions about their lives in whatever locality they live. In this chapter I consider AOP as contested practice by looking at the definition of oppression and at resistance to following through on its implications for practice. I conclude that social workers have to work in anti-oppressive ways if they are to engage and empower service users.

Defining oppression

Oppression is the devaluing of people – who they are and what they have to offer others. It is structured into social relations through the creation of binary dyads that presuppose difference and a differential evaluation of the dyad's constituent parts. For example, man-woman constitutes the 'gender' dyad; white-black a 'race' dyad; able-bodied-disabled the disabling dyad. In these binaries, one part of the dyad is ascribed superiority and the other inferiority. Those in the 'superior' group seek to organize social relations in ways that affirm their superiority in all of their traits, whether these are embedded in biology, culture or social formation. Central to this is the definition of their attributes as the 'norm' that provides the benchmark whereby others are judged. Those who are different from the norm are negatively valued or devalued as inferior. So, it is not that 'difference' is inferior, but its not being valued that makes it so.

Moreover, this difference is 'othered' to create an overall 'us-them' binary dyad that excludes those in the 'them' category. Being excluded de-legitimates their entitlement to social resources and deprives them of access to welfare provisions that are specifically identified as an entitlement of citizenship, particularly that which comes by dint of birth or acquisition through a bureaucratic process. Hence, being linked to the position of inferiority is the denial of access to various services, including employment opportunities, social services, education and health. It also includes exclusion from decision-making structures, representation on an equal basis and the right to be considered an integral and equal member of a particular territory – i.e., one who belongs. Thus, oppression becomes a structural phenomenon that can encompass any aspect of life from the spiritual to the material, from the physical to the emotional, from the personal to the sociological, political and economic.

The creation of oppressive social relations is an interactive, negotiated process that occurs as people interact with each other. Thus, no facet of living escapes the clutches of those engaging in oppressive practices. And so our understanding of oppression, if we are to successfully realize a world free of it, has to encompass its multiple dimensions, some of which we have yet to uncover and understand. Hence, oppression is more than about values. It is about power structures and social relations. Figure 8.1 indicates the holistic nature of oppression and how attempts to eradicate it have to be holistic in response. Focusing on a limited aspect of oppression might ameliorate the situation for one individual, but it will not get rid of oppression from that person's life, nor tackle the same form of oppression as it impacts on others in similar circumstances.

Oppression comes in many forms and operates on three dimensions: the personal, the institutional and the cultural. *Personal oppression* is rooted in individual beliefs, actions and behaviours. *Institutional oppression* is embedded in the policies and practices that carry social authority by being enshrined in legislation, and in policies that endorse specific kinds of goods and services as entitlements for particular types of people. These become accepted as part of everyday life and taken as routine and normal. *Cultural oppression* occurs through the values and norms that society recognizes as acceptable at a particular historical conjuncture. These are also taken as given and are therefore unlikely to be challenged or opposed by those who have a stake in social relations remaining in their current state, shaped by a rhetoric of equality, but embedded in a reality of inequalities. These three forms of oppression are interactive and feed off each other, producing a complex set of relationships that are difficult to undo easily, and are why I argue that oppression has to be dismantled in all of its aspects.

Take the instance of a policeman who stops a young black man driving a Porsche and asks him to prove that he *owns* the car, even though it has not been reported stolen (personal communication). This action contains personal racism in that the policeman does not believe that a young black man can have money (legitimately) to buy an expensive car. Thus, it must be stolen. His actions, therefore, expose taken-for-granted assumptions about ownership of expensive items, in this case linked to both class and 'race'. That this young black man and others like him are stopped on suspicions such as this one also reveals

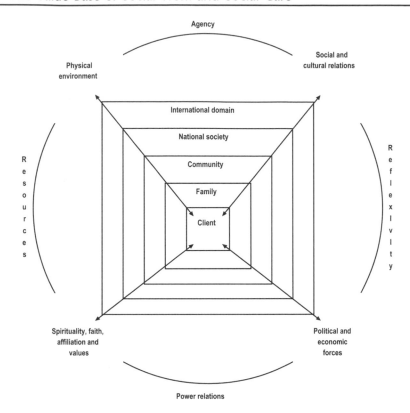

Figure 8.1 Holistic intervention for anti-oppressive practice

Source: Dominelli (2002a)

institutional racism – i.e., attitudes that have been instituted in 'stop and search' laws and actions. The policeman's personal racism and the institutional racism both draw upon cultural racism that configures young black men as thieves and trouble-makers, and as poor. Thus, racism as an oppressive social relation is reflected in its multiple, interactive and complex forms by this routine example. If the young man resists this form of surveillance and control, he is likely to be charged with other offences that may result in a court appearance, where he will be more likely to get a harsher sentence than a white person in similar circumstances. A study by the Institute of Race Relations (IRR) into the Bradford riots in 2001 found these types of dynamic in operation, with Asian defendants being given harsher sentences across the board than white defendants (IRR 2002).

Oppression is a contested term. Some people prefer to discuss structural inequalities in terms of discrimination, which for me is a much smaller part of oppression, concerned primarily with affirming equal access to social resources such as education, health services, housing, employment opportunities and political representation. Important as these are, they are not enough. Configuring oppression as discrimination fails to deal with the humiliation and attack upon a person's sense of self that is so crucial to the enactment of oppressive social relations. In addition, defining oppression as discrimination makes it easy for those who are not oppressed to deny the existence of oppression, or at best, restrict it to discrimination as practised by bigoted people. In other words, it ignores the links between structural (i.e., cultural and institutional) and personal forms of oppression. Thus, this approach fails to consider a complex web of attitudes and behaviours embedded in an inegalitarian world view that is constantly affirmed and reproduced through institutional practices, cultural norms and individual actions that treat some people as superior and others as inferior. This world view is reproduced through everyday life practices that operate on a consensual basis – i.e., they are accepted as given, or operate through violence, coercion and fear.

The dynamics of oppression

Oppressive dynamics are embedded in a world view based on the binary dyads of superiority and inferiority. A world view endorses particular ways of knowing, understanding or making sense of and experiencing society and the people within it. It also guides individuals in getting on with their lives on a daily basis. Thus, a world view is affirmed and reproduced through routine thought processes and behaviours. A world view is taken as given, and so it becomes unquestioned and the assumptions underpinning it are rarely thought about. A world view remains hegemonic or dominant as long as it is not critiqued effectively either from within or outside the dominant group. Anglocentric civilization portrays the world as having binary relations that are used to sort and categorize people and things, and privileges Anglocentric ways of organizing the world. This dyadic categorization normalizes activities or people that conform to Anglocentric norms, and by that process defines others as unacceptable. Those who do not fit this 'norm' are classified as 'deviant' people and as having a 'deficit' to make good. In racist dyads of 'black' and 'white', whiteness is privileged.

These binaries also establish the 'deserving' and 'undeserving' categorization that is used by social workers in allocating resources. The 'deserving-undeserving' binary divides clients into those who deserve assistance and those who do not. It is a crucial part of the technologies of control or 'technologies of the self' identified by Foucault (1991) as central elements in governmentality, whereby people control themselves or give their approval or consent to being controlled in particular ways. Professionals use this binary to allocate scarce resources among competing demands coming from needy people – i.e., they ration them in ways that exclude one group as possible recipients. In rationing resources, social workers prioritize some claimants as more destitute than others and end up with the following outcomes:

- Preventing some people from accessing services. In this they act as gatekeepers.
- Cutting corners to meet bureaucratic targets rather than need. In this they operate according to bureaucratic criterias of entitlement that exclude people from services they need in the name of targeting resources to the most needy and meeting performance targets.
- Providing inappropriate services, particularly by having a 'one size fits all' approach to service delivery.
- Denying individuals a real role in decision-making about the services they receive. This can become oppressive if legitimate needs are not met and people are excluded purely for bureaucratic convenience.

The many forms and multiple dimensions of oppression

Each form of oppression has its own specific characteristics. These have to be examined separately and together to alter their impact on people who are enacting such social relations, especially in situations where there is more than one form of oppression – for example, in the life of an older black lesbian. However, focusing on a particular form of oppression (e.g., racism, sexism, heterosexism, ageism, disablism) helps to better understand and address some of its unique points. A concept of converging and diverging points among different kinds of oppressive relationships helps us to consider areas that different forms of oppression have in common and elements in which they differ. This concept overcomes the difficulty of thinking in terms of hierarchies of oppression that suggest greater or lesser values to a particular type and require people who experience multiple oppressions to choose between them, rather than having all of them addressed. In other words, a person enduring multiple oppressions needs all forms of oppression to be eliminated. Additionally, multiple oppressions are interactive and are experienced simultaneously.

Convergent points or commonalities in the processes of oppression include:

- operating at all levels and interstices of everyday life;
- 'othering' people or creating dyads of inclusion and exclusion;
- normalizing some people at the expense of others;
- valuing commonalities but devaluing differences;
- denying people agency and control over their lives in the personal, institutional and cultural domains;
- reproducing inegalitarian social relations in the micro, meso and macro spheres.

Resisting oppression

The dynamics of oppression can be reproduced or resisted. Consent is required to reproduce relations of oppression. For example, reproducing an Anglocentric world view requires the active engagement of all those comprising the superior-inferior dyad as they exercise agency in conducting daily routines. Without the participation of both sides of the interactive dyad, neither its reproduction nor dominant status can be assured. The hegemonic position of a world view can be undermined or resisted by those who:

- think and act differently from accepted norms;
- reject its relevance to their lives and strike an independent path;
- challenge it with alternative visions of what can be.

Resistance can be individual or collective. However, it is difficult to turn individual acts of resistance into collective ones. For example, an individual may tell someone making offensive remarks about a black person that such behaviour is unacceptable, but this action on its own will not change the broader picture, or even prevent the same person making similar comments again. Collective resistance is needed to change a social order and promote egalitarian visions of social relations within society. There are a number of forms of resistance, and these include:

- the simple act of saying 'no';
- mass campaigns of disobedience;
- revolutionary movements.

Violence need not be an integral part of resistance. Indeed, in some situations, there is more to be lost by using violence to promote a cause rather than using non-violent means, as Ghandi's campaign of non-violence to end British rule in India demonstrated.

Poverty is a key expression of class disadvantage and remains a major source of oppression in the contemporary world. Disparities in wealth have risen within countries and between them. They have also increased dramatically during the past 20 years amidst a world of plenty and there are 1 billion people living on the absolute poverty line, defined by the United Nations (UN) as $US1 per day with a further 1.3 billion living on $US2 per day. Thus, a third of the planet's population lives below or near the absolute poverty line. Children, women-headed families and older women living alone are most affected by poverty. In neo-liberal states, the withdrawal of high quality, publicly funded services in health, housing, education and social services has had the greatest impact on poor people with reduced economic resources because they are not players on the market. They are the losers in a globalized economic world alongside the incredibly wealthy winners.

Social workers have limited scope in tackling poverty, but it affects most of the people who come to them for help. It has been sticking at about 80 per cent of service users for several decades. Securing funds that challenge the inequitable distribution of wealth is a key area for action and social workers have a crucial role to play in identifying the price that poor people pay by living in such unacceptable positions and in working with them to develop a range of strategies for tackling the problem. Such strategies vary from becoming involved in developing micro-finance schemes for poor women (Burkett 2007) to participating in anti-poverty campaigns in the international arena at the UN through its professional associations, the International Association of Schools of Social Work and the International Federation of Social Workers.

Practitioner responses to oppression

Some social work practitioners and educators find handling the complexities of oppression difficult and have little confidence in their ability to address the issues in and through their practice. Others label a concern with oppression and anti-oppression as 'political correctness' so as not to take it seriously, and can thereby justify doing nothing about it. The label of 'political correctness' is usually promulgated by those in privileged positions. It is also a response that ignores the untold suffering of those who endure oppression in myriad guises every minute of their lives. Then there are those who have struggled to empower service users and live up to the values of the profession that espouse well-being within a framework of human rights and social justice (see www.iassw-aiets.org). These individuals, black and white, have been involved in creating anti-oppressive forms of practice that place service users at the centre of a social work relationship and listen to what they have to say instead of telling them what they have to do. They seek to develop partnerships that focus on delivering appropriate services – i.e., those that take account of contexts, power relations and differential access to resources, and focus on the strengths of those that they serve. In addition, such practitioners try to change social structures that promote inequalities by demanding legislative changes and developing new forms of practice and services that involve those using them in creating, running and managing them. The services for women who had been sexually abused or subjected to male violence that feminists created as women working with women are indicative of such services (Dominelli 2002a, 2002b, 2006).

Guidelines for social work practice

Social workers can undertake a range of actions that support oppressed people's demands for a non-oppressive existence and the commitment of social resources to enhance their well-being. There is to 'tool kit' that can be prescribed to help social workers deal with the complexities of oppression. Each case should be considered in terms of its specific contexts and the agency of the person(s) concerned. There are, however, guidelines and understandings that social workers can use to help them work effectively with others to eradicate oppressive social relations. These are:

- understanding the dynamics of oppression – how it is produced and reproduced in personal thought processes or behaviours and in and through the institutional and cultural practices embedded in professional social work;
- appreciating that people are whole beings who live in specific sociopolitical and historic contexts requiring holistic interventions;
- understanding the connections between personal beliefs, institutional policies and cultural practices;
- directing efforts to eliminate oppression in all aspects of life – personal and structural – and making alliances that include those outside the profession;
- supporting claims that favour human rights and social justice.

Conclusions

Social workers have a choice. Will they continue to reproduce oppressive practices or will they work to eradicate them? If they choose the latter, they should:

- reflect upon social inequalities and take action to eradicate these on their own and, wherever possible, with others;
- be prepared for controversies that may jeopardize livelihoods;
- be proactive in ending inequalities;
- undertake research that exposes inequality of all kinds and its social construction;
- mobilize communities to challenge people's belief that oppression is an inevitable part of life;
- work towards the articulation of alternatives that are rooted in egalitarian social relations;
- form alliances with others to eliminate systemic inequalities throughout the social order.

Social workers are well placed to engage with these suggestions because they draw on skills and knowledge that they already use in their work with others. They also have the values required to make such a commitment.

References

Burkett, I. (2007) Globalised microfinance: economic empowerment or just debt? in L. Dominelli (ed.) *Revitalising Communities in a Globalising World*. Aldershot: Ashgate.

Dominelli, L. (2002a) *Anti-oppressive Social Work Theory and Practice*. London: Palgrave Macmillan.

Dominelli, L. (2002b) *Feminist Social Work Theory and Practice*. London: Palgrave Macmillan.

Dominelli, L. (2006) *Women and Community Action*. Bristol: Policy Press.

Foucault, M. (1991) Governmentality, in G. Burchell, C. Gordon and P. Miller (eds) *The Foucault Effect: Studies in Governmentality*. Hemel Hempstead: Harvester Wheatsheaf.

IRR (Institute of Race Relations) (2002) *IRR Expresses Concern over Excessive Sentencing of Bradford Rioters*, 5 July.

EXERCISE 1

The dyad

Read the following quote from Lena Dominelli:

> Oppression is the devaluing of people – who they are and what they have to offer others. It is structured into social relations through the creation of binary dyads that presuppose difference and a differential evaluation of the dyad's constituent parts. For example, man-woman constitutes the 'gender' dyad; white-black a 'race' dyad; able-bodied-disabled the disabling dyad. In these binaries, one part of the dyad is ascribed superiority and the other inferiority.

In groups, students should see how many superiority/inferiority dyads they can list in 15 minutes. How many (if any) can the groups discover where there is no inequality?

 EXERCISE 2

Students should read the following quote from Lena's chapter:

> These binaries also establish the 'deserving' and 'undeserving' categorisation that is used by social workers in allocating resources. The 'deserving-undeserving' binary divides clients into those who deserve assistance and those who do not.

Students should attempt to explore which 'categories' of service users are seen in society as 'deserving' and 'undeserving'. Take a sheet of paper, divide it down the middle and draw up two lists. What is useful and important is to identify how groups become classified as 'deserving' and 'undeserving', and why these categories have been utilized to ration resources. The following questions will be helpful in completing this exercise.

- Have these categories always been classified in this way?
- Who or what organization makes that decision?
- Are there examples where these categories have changed over the years? For example, there have been times in history

when asylum seekers were welcomed, and times when they have not been welcomed. What circumstances create such a climate?

There may also be examples where 'revelations' from research, campaigns or people speaking out have altered perceptions. Students should attempt to identify these.

 EXERCISE 3

Poverty

Students should read the section from Lena's chapter on poverty (see 'Resisting oppression', p. 121) and seek the following information:

1 What is the 'poverty line' in your country?
2 What is the 'poverty line' in the most affluent country in the world?
3 What is the 'poverty line' in the poorest country?
4 What do you think is an acceptable level of minimum income for individuals to live on in their country of origin? Does the government set such a level?

 EXERCISE 4

Promoting social justice through social work practice

Students should be invited to visit www.iassw-aiets.org and assess whether the definition of social work is adequate in relation to their country of origin.

1 If students think the definition inadequate, they should identify the shortcomings using examples drawn from practice.
2 If the definition is considered adequate, students should consider how social workers meet its claims of affirming social justice through practice, using specific examples.

chapter **nine**

ENGAGING MEN: STRATEGIES AND DILEMMAS IN VIOLENCE PREVENTION EDUCATION AMONG MEN

Michael Flood

Efforts to prevent violence against women will fail unless they undermine the cultural and collective supports for physical and sexual assault found among many men. Men are the overwhelming majority of the perpetrators of violence against women, a substantial minority of males accept violence-supportive attitudes and beliefs, and cultural constructions of masculinity shape men's use of physical and sexual violence against women. Educational strategies which lessen such social supports for violence are therefore vital. This chapter outlines recent Australian community education campaigns directed at men and the dilemmas with which they deal. It then identifies five key challenges in such work.

Violence against women is more likely in contexts in which manhood is culturally defined as linked to dominance, toughness or male honour (Heise 1998: 277). Where 'being a man' involves aggressiveness, the repression of empathy and a sense of entitlement to power, those men who are violent are acting out the dictates of what it means to be a 'normal' male. Some men are more likely to physically or sexually assault women: men who have hostile and negative sexual attitudes towards women, who identify with traditional images of masculinity and male gender role privilege, who believe in rape stereotypes, and who see violence as manly and desirable (Scully 1990; O'Neil and Harway 1997). Violence against women is more likely in families, communities, and societies that are characterized by male dominance and patriarchal authority (Heise 1998).

Violence prevention efforts must address such relationships between violence, social constructions of masculinity and gendered power relations. Formal prevention and control strategies such as sound laws and integrated criminal responses are important. They can help victims' recovery and hinder perpetrators' reoffending, and they have symbolic value. But they can do little in a climate where most women do not formally report abusive events, where most survivors remain silent (DeKeseredy *et al.* 2000: 921), and where dominant beliefs about violence convince many women that their experience was not rape or assault at all or that it was *their* fault (Kelly and Radford 1996).

Men have been invited to contribute to the goal of ending violence against women in various contexts: in perpetrator programmes, through pro-feminist men's anti-violence activism (Flood 2005), through education in the police, law and medicine, and through community education campaigns. The remainder of this chapter centres on the last approach. I focus on efforts directed at adult men rather than those directed at boys (e.g. in schools), although many of the dilemmas discussed are similar.

There is in most western countries a systematic gender gap in attitudes towards violence (Flood and Pease 2006). A significant minority of males agree with violence-supportive beliefs and myths, and males continue to show more violence-supportive attitudes than females. In Australia for example, the most recent national survey found that a fifth of men agreed that 'Women often say "No" when they mean "Yes" ', and a sixth agreed that 'Women who are raped often ask for it' (ANOP Research Services 1995). One in six males aged between 12 and 20 agreed that 'It's okay for a boy to make a girl have sex with him if she has flirted with him or led him on' (see National Crime Prevention 2001: 64–70). In general, males have narrower definitions of domestic violence than females and they are less likely to rate a range of forms of violence as very serious. At the same time, men's (and women's) attitudes are improving over time.

Violence prevention

In Australia only a handful of community education campaigns have attempted to undermine social and cultural supports among adult men for violence against women. However, a relatively recent New South Wales (NSW) campaign is one of the best examples of community education directed at men. The campaign was called 'Violence Against Women — It's Against All the Rules', and was run from 2000 to 2003 by the Violence Against Women Specialist Unit of the NSW Attorney General's Department. The campaign was targeted at men aged 21 to 29, and took the form of posters, booklets and radio advertisements. It used high profile sportsmen and sporting language to deliver the message that violence against women is unacceptable. For example, a famous rugby league player was shown alongside the words, 'Force a woman into touch? That's sexual assault'. A well-known cricketer said, 'Sledging a woman? That's abuse'. A soccer player said, 'Mark a woman, watch her every move? That's stalking'.

Defining manhood as non-violent

Community education strategies directed at men have adopted three broad approaches. The first is to promote alternative constructions of masculinity, gender and selfhood which foster non-violence. This embodies the recognition that men's violence against women is informed by the cultural association between violence and masculinity – by the social construction of violence as a normal, palatable or inevitable part of manhood. Some campaigns enact this strategy indirectly. The NSW campaign tried to rewrite the cultural meanings given to men's violent behaviour, by linking physical and sexual behaviours to actions on the sporting field which are literally 'against the rules'. Other campaigns have tried more directly to re-script cultural expectations of manhood or undermine an association between manhood and violence.

Efforts to lessen men's tolerance of violence against women at times have attempted to redefine violence as unmanly or manliness as non-violent, therefore representing violence and masculinity as contradictory. 'Real men don't bash or rape women' was the bold message of some posters in the 1993–4 national campaign conducted by the Office for the Status of Women. Similarly, the NSW campaign materials stated that 'sports role models can show that a masculine man is not a violent man' (Violence Against Women Specialist Unit 2000: 24). Although the notion of redefining masculinity as non-violent was not explicit in the NSW advertisements, a quarter of men who encountered the campaign described the main message as being, 'You don't have to be violent to be a real man' (see Hubert 2003: 38–9).

Community education campaigns overseas have used similar strategies. The American campaign 'My strength is not for hurting' encouraged men to practise consent and respect in their sexual relations. This campaign attempted to reconfigure a trait traditionally associated with masculinity – strength – such that it embodied non-violence and moral selfhood. Other approaches ask, 'Are you *man enough* to turn away from violence [or] to stand up to violence?', or describe violence as 'weak' and 'cowardly'. The first draws upon boys' existing investments in male identity and their desires to become adult men, in order to invite non-violence, while the second represents violence as contrary to the qualities of strength, bravery, self-control and moral courage associated with 'true' masculinity (Gilbert and Gilbert 1998: 247). Such approaches represent a strategy of both complicity in and challenge to masculinity. On the one hand, appeals to male identity and stereotypically masculine qualities are complicit in common constructions of masculinity and collude with males' investments in manhood. On the other hand, such appeals also attempt to shift the meanings associated with maleness.

We should be wary of approaches which appeal to men's sense of 'real' manhood or invite them to 'prove themselves *as men*'. These may intensify men's investment in male identity, and this is part of what keeps patriarchy in place (Stoltenberg 1990). Such appeals are especially problematic if they suggest that there are particular qualities which are essentially or exclusively male. This reinforces notions of biological essentialism and determinism and denies valuable qualities, such as strength and courage, to women. Nevertheless, community education addressing males should speak to questions of identity. Boys and young men often struggle with the formation of their gendered identities, negotiating competing discourses of manhood and heterosexuality. There is often a dichotomy between their public projection of a confident masculinity and their experience of private anxieties and insecurities (Mac an Ghaill 1994: 99). These processes of identity formation represent a critical opportunity for violence prevention. Education campaigns can model identities based on moral reasoning, justice and selfhood rather than gender-identity anxiety, dominance and manhood (Stoltenberg 2001).

A strategy of complicity and challenge is an understandable and indeed desirable response to the real challenge of educating men on gender issues. Efforts to reach men must negotiate a tension between two necessary elements: between speaking to men in ways which engage with the realities of their lives, and transforming the patriarchal power relations and gendered discourses which are the fabric of those same lives.

Drawing on masculine culture

It is now firmly established in violence prevention networks that one's strategies must be 'culturally appropriate'. They must be sensitive to the audience's values and needs and draw on culturally-specific languages. The NSW campaign's use of sporting language is an ideal example, and evaluations suggest that men did perceive the campaign as meaningful and clever.

However, there is little discourse among men with which to build a culture of violence prevention, and this poses real difficulties for community education. The NSW campaign was unsuccessful in encouraging men to talk about violence against women. Ninety per cent of men in the target group who had seen or heard something of the campaign reported that violence against women was not an issue they would talk about with their peers (Hubert 2003: 32–3). Aboriginal men were the exception, and this reflects a growing conversation in indigenous communities about family violence and sexual abuse.

In trying to appeal to and engage with men, education campaigns have drawn on stereotypical masculine culture. This poses more fundamental dilemmas for violence prevention. The NSW campaign drew on male-focused sports, but sporting culture also contributes to the construction of violent masculinity as a cultural norm. Sport is an important site for teaching boys and men some of the key values associated with dominant masculinity, such as extreme competitiveness, aggression and dominance. The 'combat sport subculture' of games such as rugby melds athleticism, manliness and violence (Schissel 2000). Violence is normalized, naturalized and rewarded in sport (Messner 1992). Also, athletes report significantly greater agreement with rape-supportive statements than men in general (Boeringer 1999), and cultures of misogyny have been documented in hockey (West 1996; Robinson 1998) and rugby (Schacht 1996). To be fair, the NSW campaign may have addressed these issues by simultaneously shifting sporting culture as it shifts the attitudes of men in general, in that the campaign involved sporting clubs, training of sportsmen as educators and sports sponsorship.

This example illustrates the dilemmas in drawing on masculine culture to reach men. Approaches such as those in the NSW campaign and the American 'My strength is not for hurting' campaign represent a difficult balancing act between complicity and challenge. They collude enough with masculine cultural codes that they engage a male audience, yet hopefully they subvert the association of masculinity and violence enough to make a difference to men's attitudes and behaviours.

Men speaking out

The third key strategy in community education campaigns directed at men is to show men speaking out or standing together against violence. Some campaigns use male celebrities and sporting heroes in their materials, while others depict 'ordinary' men of the community collectively voicing their concern about violence against women.

There are three rationales for this strategy. First, these men function as role models, whose intolerance of violence ideally will be emulated. Focus group participants for the NSW campaign perceived the sportsmen to be credible and authoritative 'real men'. But they also praised the fact that these were 'ordinary blokes' with faults and weaknesses, rather than 'gods' like Pat Rafter who probably 'unpacks the dishwasher for his mum' (see Hubert 2003: 40–1). Second, peer acceptance and collective norms are particularly influential among men. Men's lives are highly organized by relations between men. Males seek the approval of other males, both identifying with and competing against them. If men's perceptions of collective masculine norms can be shifted, then individual men may shift as well. Third, ours is a culture in which men's voices are granted greater authority than women's voices. It is probably true that men will listen more to men than to women. We may think it highly desirable that men listen to *women's* voices, to women's stories of the harms and indeed the pleasures of their relations with men. But it may be more effective to continue to use men to say the things that we wish men could hear from women.

Key challenges

In violence prevention work with males, the overarching challenge is to both engage with and reconstruct men and masculine culture. There are five further challenges in this work.

Undermine discourses of sexuality

The first challenge is to undermine powerful discourses of masculinity and heterosexuality which support violence against women. For example, some men (and women) subscribe to the idea that male sexuality is an uncontrollable or barely controllable force or 'drive' (Kippax *et al.* 1994: S318). This notion has been used to deny, downplay or defend men's sexual violence against women, and to place the burden of responsibility for rape with women. It is up to women not to 'provoke' men or 'lead them on', as men cannot be held responsible for their actions (Richardson 1997: 161). Such notions are related to a second discourse in which women are the gatekeepers and guardians of sexual safety, with responsibility for both their own and men's sexual behaviour.

A third construction, the sexual double standard, also feeds into sexual violence. This involves two standards of sexual behaviour: girls and women who are sexually active or seen to be so receive negative sexual reputations as 'sluts' or 'slags' (or any of a wide variety of other terms), while males receive positive labels like 'stud' or 'legend'. More widely, women's sexual behaviour is highly controlled and harshly judged, while men's sexual behaviour is freer of social constraint (Holland *et al.* 1996; Hillier *et al.* 1998). Rape is often excused or denied with reference to women as 'sluts', and young women perceived as 'easy' are likely to be more vulnerable to sexual violence (National Crime Prevention 2001: 43). These constructions must be eroded, through innovative and culturally relevant messages.

Teach young men how to do consent

In running workshops with young heterosexual men, I have asked, 'How do you know that you are not pressuring the girl you're with into sex?' (Flood 2002). Many young men rely on problematic indicators such as the absence of resistance, body language, or previous or current sexual activity. Many have little idea of how to negotiate different forms of sexual activity and are too embarrassed or self-conscious to explicitly negotiate consent. And indeed, some young men simply do not care whether or not the girl is consenting, or even find forced sex arousing. It is vital that we teach young men why consent is important *and* how to negotiate it.

Target masculine bonding and culture

Male bonding feeds sexual violence against women, and sexual violence against women feeds male bonding. The cultures and collective rituals of male bonding among closely knit male fraternities, street gangs and male athletes foster the sexual assault of women (Martin and Hummer 1989; Sanday 1990). In turn, rape can be practised as a means to and an expression of male bonding (Scully 1990). Especially among young men, attachment to male peers who encourage and legitimate woman abuse is a significant predictor of perpetrating abuse (Flood and Pease 2006: 40–2).

Violence prevention strategies among men must therefore also include interventions into local violence-supportive cultures. On university campuses with high rates of sexual violence, some of the sociocultural correlates (especially among male college fraternities) include an ethic of male sexual conquest, high alcohol consumption, homophobia, use of pornography and general sexist norms (Sanday 1996).

Address social diversity

Prevention strategies must also address the complex intersections of class, race and ethnicity which shape women's and men's experiences of and involvements in assault. For example, male perpetrators are more likely to be held accountable and criminalized, and their crimes are more likely to be seen as linked to their ethnicity, if they are poor, black or men of colour (Russo 2001: 147–62).

Is it possible to acknowledge that males' violence-supportive attitudes are shaped by social variables such as ethnicity without also reinforcing racism? A recent national survey found that among young people aged 12 to 20, about a fifth agreed with the use of violence by both sexes. These young people were more likely to be male, younger (12–14 years), of lower socioeconomic status, and from Middle Eastern or Asian backgrounds. This cluster was also significantly more likely to hold traditional views about gender roles (National Crime Prevention 2001: 81–90).

The ease with which existing racist assumptions can be reinforced was illustrated in the experience of the NSW campaign. While more than half of men correctly perceived that the campaign was aimed at men in general, one in eight thought it was aimed at particular ethnic groups (Hubert 2003: 36–7).

Address men's victimization

The final challenge, perhaps the hardest of them all, is to address men's own experience of violence and to preempt the rejection of violence prevention messages associated with not doing so. In evaluations of the NSW campaign, some men responded that men too are the victims of violence, including by women (Hubert 2003: 50–1).

There are three ways of understanding this complaint. Perhaps it is a legitimate claim about men's own subjection to violence, as men are the majority of the victims of physical assaults and homicide. But the great majority of perpetrators are also male. Men are most at risk of physical harm from other men, whereas the men in the NSW campaign who emphasized men's victimization seemed to focus on violence *by women*.

This leads to a second explanation, in which this response is an expression of anti-feminist backlash and defensiveness. It represents the success of men's rights and fathers' rights advocates in communicating the falsehood that women are violent to men as much as men are violent to women. (For critiques of this claim, see Flood 1999 and Kimmel 2002.) And it is a defensive reaction to the critique of men's violence against women.

However, in a third reading, this response is an inevitable although misleading extension of feminist successes in redefining violence. Feminist accounts of domestic violence routinely list verbal, emotional and psychological forms of abuse alongside physical violence. These embody the recognition that men's physical violence to women is very often accompanied by other forms of abusive and harmful behaviour (Macdonald 1998: 27–32). But they also allow men to rename their own experiences of verbal conflict, name-calling, and stereotypically feminine 'nagging' as 'verbal and emotional abuse' or 'emotional violence'. In many cases, this trivializes the term 'violence' by applying it to instances of their female partners' behaviour which are unpleasant but not particularly harmful. It also represents an ignorance of the real horror associated with the systematic emotional and psychological abuse to which some women are subjected. Whichever reading we think is most accurate, we will need to respond to men's perceptions of victimization.

Conclusion

Profound changes in men's lives and social constructions of masculinity are necessary if violence against women is to be eliminated. Community education strategies are a key element in violence prevention. They face particular challenges when they are addressed, as they must be, to men.

Acknowledgement

A version of this chapter was first published in *Women Against Violence*, 13, 2002–3 (Melbourne: CASA House).

References

ANOP Research Services (1995) *Community Attitudes to Violence Against Women: Detailed Report*. Canberra: Department of the Prime Minister and Cabinet, Office of the Status of Women.

Boeringer, S.B. (1999) Associations of rape-supportive attitudes with fraternal and athletic participation, *Violence Against Women*, 5(1): 81–90.

DeKeseredy, W.S., Schwartz, M.D. and Alvi, S. (2000) The role of pro-feminist men in dealing with woman abuse on the Canadian college campus, *Violence Against Women*, 6(9): 918–35.

Flood, M. (1999) Claims about husband battering, *DVIRC Newsletter*, summer: 3–8.

Flood, M. (2002) Tips for good sex workshop. Unpublished.

Flood, M. (2005) Men's collective struggles for gender justice: the case of anti-violence activism, in M. Kimmel, J. Hearn and R.W. Connell (eds) *The Handbook of Studies on Men and Masculinities*. Thousand Oaks, CA: Sage.

Flood, M. and Pease, P. (2006) *The Factors Influencing Community Attitudes in Relation to Violence Against Women: A Critical Review of the Literature*. Melbourne: Victorian Health Promotion Foundation.

Gilbert, R. and Gilbert, P. (1998) *Masculinity Goes to School*. Sydney: Allen & Unwin.

Heise, L. (1998) Violence against women: an integrated, ecological framework, *Violence Against Women*, 4(3): 262–83.

Hillier, L., Harrison, L. and Warr, D. (1998) 'When you carry condoms all the boys think you want it': negotiating competing discourses about safe sex, *Journal of Adolescence*, 21(1): 15–29.

Holland, J., Ramazanoglu, C., Sharpe, S. and Thomson, R. (1996) Reputations: journeying into gendered power relations, in J. Weeks and J. Holland (eds) *Sexual Cultures: Communities, Values and Intimacy*. Basingstoke: Macmillan.

Hubert, C. (2003) *Violence Against Women: It's Against All the Rules – Evaluation of the NSW Statewide Campaign to Reduce Violence Against Women*. Sydney: Violence Against Women Specialist Unit, NSW Attorney General's Department.

Kelly, L. and Radford, J. (1996) 'Nothing really happened': the invalidation of women's experiences of sexual violence, in M. Hester, L. Kelly and J. Radford (eds) *Women, Violence and Male Power*. Buckingham: Open University Press.

Kimmel, M.S. (2002) 'Gender symmetry' in domestic violence: a substantive and methodological research review, *Violence Against Women*, 8(11): 1332–63.

Kippax, S., Crawford, J. and Waldby, C. (1994) Heterosexuality, masculinity and HIV, *AIDS*, 8(suppl. 1): S315–23.

Mac an Ghaill, M. (1994) *The Making of Men: Masculinities, Sexualities and Schooling*. Buckingham: Open University Press.

Macdonald, H (1998) *What's in a Name? Definitions and Domestic Violence*. Brunswick, VIC: Domestic Violence and Incest Resource Centre.

Martin, P. and Hummer, R. (1989) Fraternities and rape on campus, *Gender and Society*, 3(4): 457–73.

Messner, M.A. (1992) When bodies are weapons, *Peace Review*, 4(3): 28–31.

National Crime Prevention (2001) *Young People and Domestic Violence: National Research on Young People's Attitudes and Experiences of Domestic Violence*. Canberra: Crime Prevention Branch, Commonwealth Attorney-General's Department.

O'Neil, J. and Harway, M. (1997) A multivariate model explaining men's violence toward women: predisposing and triggering hypotheses, *Violence Against Women*, 3(2): 182–203.

Richardson, D. (1997) Sexuality and feminism, in V. Robinson and D. Richardson (eds) *Introducing Women's Studies: Feminist Theory and Practice*. Basingstoke: Macmillan.

Robinson, L. (1998) *Crossing the Line: Violence and Sexual Assault in Canada's National Sport*. Toronto: McLelland & Stewart.

Russo, A. (2001) *Taking Back Our Lives: A Call to Action for the Violence Against Women Movement*. New York: Routledge.

Sanday, P. (1990) *Fraternity Gang Rape: Sex, Brotherhood, and Privilege on Campus*. New York: New York University Press.

Sanday, P. (1996) Rape-prone versus rape-free campus cultures, *Violence Against Women*, 2(2): 191–208.

Schacht, S. (1996) Misogyny on and off the 'pitch': the gendered world of male rugby players, *Gender & Society*, 10(5): 550–65.

Schissel, B. (2000) Boys against girls: the structural and interpersonal dimensions of violent patriarchal culture in the lives of young men, *Violence Against Women*, 6(9): 960–86.

Scully, D. (1990) *Understanding Sexual Violence: A Study of Convicted Rapists*. Boston, MA: Unwin Hyman.

Stoltenberg, J. (1990) *Refusing to be a Man: Essays on Sex and Justice*. London: Fontana/Collins.

Stoltenberg, J. (2001) Re: [PROFEM] men can stop rape. *Profem Discussion List* (online), 5 February, profem-l@coombs.anu.edu.au.

Violence Against Women Specialist Unit (2000) *Violence Against Women — It's Against All the Rules*. Sydney: NSW Attorney General's Department.

West, W.G. (1996) Youth sports and violence: a masculine subculture? in G. O'Bireck (ed.) *Not a Kid Anymore: Canadian Youth, Crime, and Subcultures*. Toronto: Nelson.

EXERCISE 1

What do know about violence and abuse in your country?

> The task is to obtain the most up-to-date information about violence and abuse in your country. Students should be divided into several groups to undertake project work:
>
> - In your country, who or what organizations first began to express concern about domestic violence? Students should trace back to the beginnings of safe houses for women and children suffering violence.
> - What reports first became known and in which professions?
> - Was there a 'movement' against violence and abuse?
> - What organizations challenged the notion of there being a problem?

 EXERCISE 2

Where is violence and abuse to women and children most prevalent in the world?

> Students should examine international reports and find out whether there are similarities or differences between nation states regarding violence and abuse. Students can divide into sub-groups and be allotted a country to examine. A range of countries can be chosen. Information can be gathered from many sources (e.g. United Nations reports, non-governmental organizations, academic papers, pressure groups etc.).
> Students should then consider Michael Flood's comment:
>
> > Violence against women is more likely in contexts in which manhood is culturally defined as linked to dominance, toughness or male honour.
>
> Students should be encouraged to consider this comment and examine the country concerned in relation to the following questions:
>
> - How does that country represent gender relations?

- In what ways does the culture of that country accept or challenge the behaviour of men?
- What research is there in that country on violence and abuse?
- Is there a 'robust' legal system to deal with men's violence?
- Are there (at the time that this exercise is being undertaken) any campaigns to inform public opinion?

Students may want to draw up a system of clarifying what each country has – perhaps a grid of key points. When completed, students can use this as a source of discussion and debate.

 EXERCISE 3

Developing a campaign to change violent male behaviour

This is an exciting and potentially productive task where students as a group can undertake some work which will help make a difference in a town, city or community. Before the work is undertaken the facilitator needs to undertake the groundwork with a range of agencies who are involved in violence and abuse prevention, based in the areas the students would like to undertake the project. Most areas now have domestic violence forums, and diplomacy is absolutely *critical*, as are negotiation, advanced warning, agreement and collaboration. Much of this groundwork needs to be done by the university, trainer or facilitator well before students become active on a project.

Stage 1

Groundwork with key agencies – communicate what you would like to do, explain the learning objectives, try to be useful to services which are normally overstretched.

Stage 2

Students should explore:

- What sort of campaign could be run 'locally' to explore how to challenge men's violence.
- What would that campaign look like?

- Is there any evidence that such campaigns help reduce men's violence?
- What local agencies should take the lead or be a part of this?

Students could develop a project group and liaise with a range of services and agencies to obtain help. If this is just a 'paper exercise' then there may not be as much need to make contacts. However, this could be a project where participants can help contribute to promote important issues. Students could liaise with local practitioners, legal services, law enforcement services, publicans and breweries in order to develop a project which could come to fruition at the end of an academic term. Hard-pressed voluntary services could benefit from this input.

The facilitator should hold this all together, as students working without guidelines or support could easily fail.

chapter **ten**

SOCIAL WORK AND MANAGEMENT

Ray Jones

When I attended a large conference of over 300 people on a radical agenda for social work at Liverpool University in 2006, I was the only (as far as I know) senior social services manager present. When I introduced myself as a social services director before making a comment in one of the plenary sessions, about half of the audience booed (I had a similar hostile reception from some delegates when speaking at the Unison National Social Services Conference in 2005). This was followed by some sympathetic and supportive applause from others. The comment I went on to make was about the importance of building joint agendas – shaped by service users – between practitioners, managers and policy-makers based on the value base of social work!

So, is it possible to uphold the values of social work in management roles? What are these values anyway? And is it necessary and inevitable that there should be a distance, and indeed some distaste, between social workers as practitioners and managers (many of whom still hold as a part of their primary identity that they are social workers)?

Management

First of all, what is this thing called 'management'? Well it is not something only or usually done by 'the boss'. It involves us all. We are all managers. Power, however, is not evenly distributed and position status, 'being a manager', has more formal organizational power allocated to it than 'being a social worker' within the organization. But, as argued by Veronica Coulshed (and developed in Coulshed *et al.* 2006), 'all social workers are managers. Their circles of activity ripple outwards from managing themselves, at the core, to managing others, and onwards again to managing systems'. These are all themes to which we will return, and they are reiterated by Martin and Henderson (2001: 22) who write about management encompassing 'managing people, managing activities, managing resources, managing information, and doing all these through managing self'.

There is also a difference to be noted between 'management' and 'leadership', and indeed today 'leadership' is often more topical than 'management'. This partly reflects differences in understanding and emphasis in how we conceptualize organizations and interactions – the concept of mechanistic, structured bureaucracies contrasting with organic, reflective systems.

With the advent of social services departments in the 1970s there was a flurry of activity, supported by social services' own organizational think-tank at Brunel University (see BIOSS 1974, 1980), with hierarchical structure charts being drawn to illustrate how staff might be deployed and harnessed together within work groups, how resources would be allocated (downwards through the structure) and how accountability would be achieved (usually upwards) through line management relationships.

Managers have since drawn similar structure charts to picture and describe the new organizational arrangements developed to meet changing requirements and differing views about how best to organize social care (such as the localization rather than centralization of services; the specialist separation into children's and adult services rather than generic teams; the integration of social workers within multidisciplinary teams with the National Health Service (NHS) or with other children's services; or the advent of strategic planning, commissioning, service purchasing and care management discrete from the direct delivery and provision of services). All of these changes were based on new wisdoms to tackle perceived current difficulties, but rarely has their impact been properly assessed and usually the changes were never piloted but were a 'big bang' response to new political imperatives or changing organizational and management fashion.

The chaos which can be caused by too frequent and poorly managed change is well illustrated by the current state of the NHS, where politically driven manic agendas lead to continuous disruption which is never given time to settle down to see if the changes will deliver the gains intended. The consequence is confusion about organizational values and goals, and a workforce which experiences 'macho management', with managers themselves feeling vulnerable within a culture of harassment and threat.

This can be contrasted with a focus on organizations as organic systems with formal and informal cultures, recognizing that relationships are the medium for much activity, that motivation and morale are key in setting and delivering a vision and direction, with learning and feeding back being central to performance, and with an emphasis on leadership as well as (but not instead of) management.

Management might be seen as 'keeping the show on the road', seeking to ensure that resources are appropriately allocated and properly managed, and that performance targets are set and achieved. This is more than 'administration', which is the term which had been used to describe what we now see as 'management' (note that we still have Masters in Business Administration, MBA, degrees, although we no longer have 'health service administrators' heading up hospitals and other NHS organizations). Administrators have their own expertise in developing and maintaining processes and procedures within organizations. Managers have a responsibility and accountability for the organization's use of resources and overall performance.

Leadership

But what about 'leaders'? Leadership is about setting, hopefully in partnership with others, the direction for the organization, painting a picture, a vision, of what could be, and how this could be better, as well as having a concern for current performance (both because of its immediate impact and because it is the platform for moving forward).

Hartley and Allison (2003), when discussing 'leadership', look at the leader as a 'person', with a focus on their skills, abilities, personality, styles and behaviour (which can often be impacted by opportunity and the situation – such as the response and profile of Mayor Giuliani in New York after 9/11). They then look at their 'position', which refers to a formal position in an organization such as a team leader or chief executive, and then at the 'process', which focuses on the dynamics within an organization and between people.

Hartley and Allison note that with regard to leadership as a process, 'leadership is concerned with motivating and influencing people, and shaping and achieving outcomes' (2003: 298). They then go on to describe two types of leadership, first conceptualized by Burns (1978). 'Transactional leadership' is about overseeing how an organization works by establishing mechanisms and processes to achieve current goals. 'Transformational leadership' is about seeing possibilities beyond the present, setting a vision, mapping a route forward and motivating others through the process of change.

Hartley and Allison refer to Nadler and Tushman (1989), who describe 'transformational leadership' as 'envisioning', 'energizing' and 'enabling'. To these 'Es' could be added the 'Es' of 'exciting' and 'enthusing' as a means of creating commitment. As Adair (2006: 34) notes: 'Enthusiasm, integrity, the combination of toughness and demandingness and fairness, humanity and warmth, humility (openness and lack of arrogance); these are some of the generic qualities of a good leader – and a leader for good'.

'Transactional', rather than 'transformational' leadership can be related to the focus of government public sector policy over recent decades. The Thatcher and subsequent Conservative governments in the UK emphasized the three 'Es' (more 'Es'!) of economy, efficiency and effectiveness (and occasionally another 'E' of 'equity') for public sector organizations, focusing on 'value for money', with competition within a market of services and providers to drive improved performance and responsiveness for service users. This could be described as 'transactional leadership', and there was certainly a very high concern for the processes and structures within public sector organizations, which resulted in, for example, a 'purchaser-provider' separation (see e.g. Butt and Palmer 1985; Flynn 1990; for a more critical comment see Holman 1993).

However, in the context of tight restraints on public sector expenditure (except, unintentionally, escalating social security payments to the numbers of unemployed people, which soared under Thatcher), the focus on the three 'Es' gave management within social work a bad (or should it be worse!) name:

> managerialism promised that the state goals could be attained with the use of fewer resources. The revitalising of managers was seen as the key to achieving this ambitious 'more for less' agenda ... managers' alleged underperformance was to be addressed through the incorporation into social work of management practices from the private sector in order to revitalise and equip it for a new challenge ... by such means, those seen previously as professionally tainted [as social workers] were to be turned into uncontaminated activist managers.
>
> (Harris 2003: 47)

It also had an impact on the position of women within management:

> The deep recession of 1989/94, Government reforms, and technological developments forced a dramatic change throughout the private and public employment sectors. De-layering, re-structuring, down-sizing, and being more bottom-line conscious caused a flood of side-effects. Managers found themselves rafting down white water.

The best managers went on developing and training their staff and pursuing their equal opportunities policies, but many line managers under pressure to meet tight budget margins for competitive tendering often cut back on such 'luxury extras'. Worse, the practical outcome of de-layering has often been to abolish the upper limits of employment women had just reached, squeezing them out.

(Abdela 1995: 8)

And, as Abdela had previously noted, this came on top of the barriers already being experienced by women and other 'minorities':

The undeniable fact is in the vast majority of United Kingdom organisations the environment, work systems and structures have been Savile Row tailor-made to suit mainly white males with few direct responsibilities for caring for children or other relatives at home. The ways in which careers develop, the mobility required of senior staff, often the need to have international experience and formal qualifications, the networks, all absolutely rest upon the viewpoint and perceptions of a male world. 'Minorities' like women, ethnic groups and the disabled have always been required to work within systems and work cultures designed precisely to suit the needs and customs of a completely different group of people.

(Abdela 1991: 4)

This is a dynamic which continues, as noted more recently by Flood and Pease (2005: 121): 'Unjust gender relations are maintained by individual men's sexist and gendered practices, masculine workplace cultures, men's monopolies over decision-making and leadership, and powerful constructions of masculine and male identity'.

There has been some policy and legislative progress since the mid-1990s to address some of the issues which have discriminated against and disadvantaged women, people from an ethnic or cultural minority, or disabled people (and also men wanting to be more engaged as parents and carers), but with regard to the government's approach to the public sector, 'New Labour' since 1997 has continued the focus on 'transactional management' (indeed to the extent that it has become micro-management of local activity by central government and its civil service), with increased attention being given to processes, procedures and performance within public sector organizations.

This has been achieved through the deployment of strengthened inspectorates (such as the Commission for Social Care Inspection within social care in England, and similar inspectorates in the other UK nations, but also the Healthcare Commission and Ofsted) and the public reports and ratings of how organizations are managed and are performing.

Indeed, New Labour have invented and deployed a new armoury of means to get public sector organizations to change in line with central government wishes, and these can be described as the six 'Ms' of political transactional micro-management:

1 *Management by machismo:* achieving an impact through threat and fear, such as directors of 'failing' social services authorities being called up to London to meet with the social services chief inspector and with their jobs on the line.
2 *Management by message:* with clusters of performance indicators and national policy statements indicating where attention should be given.
3 *Management by measurement:* what gets measured gets done!
4 *Management by motivation:* with rewards (performance stars and honours) for achievements, and punishments (monthly visits by inspectors) for failures.
5 *Management by money:* with government-specific grants determining what and how services should be developed.
6 *Management by mistake:* the unintended consequences which sometimes occur, such as the government's performance target on how much assistance a local council provides excluding the spend on voluntary sector and community development, with this expenditure then deterred as it does not assist the performance rating.

As Jordan and Jordan (2000: 84) comment: 'the principles of [New Labour's] "third way" outline a programme of modernisation by means of a characteristically Benthamite, regulatory and supervisory method, with the threat of heavy penalties for non-compliance'.

However, it could also be argued that the New Labour public service 'modernization' agenda (see e.g. Department of Health 1998) is also in some ways 'transformational', with its vision of a new role for the public sector – what might be characterized as a fourth 'E' of 'empowering'. This is described as being about contestability (a New Labour word for Thatcher's competition) across services, but also about increased user choice and control through, for example, direct payments and individual budgets.

This also now includes recognizing people's capacity, competence and contribution as citizens, rather than an overwhelming focus on delivering services and providing assistance to tackle the problems of people and places, of individuals and communities.

For social care in England (and again with similarities in the other UK nations), this new 'empowering agenda' for public services has been further shaped by the White Paper *Every Child Matters* (Department for Education and Skills 2003), by the social care government Green Paper for adults, *Independence, Well-being and Choice* (Department of Health 2005) and by the government's health and social care White Paper, *Our Health, Our Care, Our Say* (Department of Health 2006). However, in the absence of an adequate allocation of resources (money and time) to assist people who are disadvantaged and deprived, or distressed and disturbed, the 'empowering agenda' can become an euphemism for 'benign neglect'.

While escaping the paternalistic and patronizing attitudes (doing 'to' and 'for' rather than 'with' or 'by' people) which have been inherent within some areas of social care, the empowerment agenda still means that in reality people without their own immediate means to purchase assistance are left stranded without help or receive second-rate, poor-quality services (such as being on a waiting list for a care home and and then ending up with a shared room, or receiving very heavily rationed and restricted home care services).

Social work's value base

Having reflected above more generally on management and leadership, and on social work and social care management within changing political contexts, what about the relationship between the value base of social work and management?

Firstly, some comment on the value base of social work. There is a strong historical track record of social work proclaiming and re-emphasizing its value base (see e.g., from each decade in the past 50 years, Biestek 1961; British Association of Social Workers 1977; Barclay Report 1982; Bamford 1990; Gilroy 2004), which can be summarized as:

- having a concern for social justice;
- confronting discrimination;

- valuing people and not rejecting them, but with realism as well as idealism;
- seeing people in context;
- recognizing and developing people's strengths and skills;
- problem-solving in partnership;
- enabling and facilitating, with a focus on relationships;
- providing structure and space within chaotic experiences;
- being an ally in promoting independence and choice;
- developing and harnessing resources;
- not running away from pain;
- taking actions to protect and control where necessary.

This has all been reinforced by recent government and government-commissioned reports in Scotland (Scottish Executive 2006), Wales (Welsh Assembly 2006) and England (GSCC 2007) and all draws on and fits within the International Federation of Social Workers' definition of social work, which states:

> The social work profession promotes social change, problem-solving in human relationships and the empowerment and liberation of people to enhance well-being. Using theories of human behaviour and social systems, social work intervenes at the points where people interact with their environments. Principles of human rights and social justice are fundamental to social work.
>
> (International Federation of Social Workers 2000)

So, how and to what extent can social work's value base provide a platform for good management, and are the values of social work sustainable as practitioners move into management roles?

Social work and management: some thoughts

Social workers could and should make good managers. This is because, firstly, management and leadership require emotional intelligence as well as intellectual intelligence. This is explored by Goleman *et al.* (2002), and builds on Goleman's earlier writing on emotional intelligence (Goleman 1996). If social workers are competent at assessing people and their social situations, and are skilled in building and using relationships to achieve intended outcomes, then these are all competencies which are of immediate relevance to good management, as is the ability and confidence to confront difficult and challenging behaviours and issues.

It is also of importance for good management to be able to build and harness resources to achieve goals, and the social planning (see Barclay Report 1982) and political and systems management skills of social workers are of relevance here.

Secondly, the conceptual and theoretical underpinnings of social work practice are also relevant to management. Problem-solving approaches, task-centred models, cognitive therapy and learning theories, approaches to understanding community inter-actions and community development, systems analysis and sys-tems management, can all on reflection be seen to have lessons for good management practice and behaviours.

Put all of this alongside, thirdly, the values of social work, which are about promoting justice and fairness, and tackling discrimination and – fourthly – noting the skills of social workers in conflict identification and resolution, then it becomes clear that social workers certainly should take a very relevant batch of understandings and competencies into management roles.

But this does require some re-setting of personal and profes-sional identities. Being a paid manager within an organization is not the same as being a more highly paid social worker, although it would be very positive if social workers did not have to move up through management hierarchies for occupational and career progression, and this is recognized in the recent General Social Care Council (GSCC) (2007) report.

The roles are different, and managers have particular respon-sibilities and accountabilities for the deployment and use of resources such as worker time and budgets, and for overall performance, which does require from time to time confronting and tackling poor performance. But the need to stay credible as a manager and leader, and to continue to uphold the value base of social work, requires being human, keeping informed, being honest, and managing role conflicts and tensions.

'Being human' means not distancing oneself from the pain and difficulties being experienced by others, be they service users or colleagues, and acknowledging distress. It also means being 'out there' when the going gets tough and when, as is bound to happen from time to time, there is a dramatic event such as a child being seriously injured or dying, or a disabled or older person being stranded without the essential assistance they re-quire.

Organizations often speak about a 'no blame culture' and being a 'learning organization'. For managers this should mean being close to front-line staff and being recognized as understand-ing the realities, including the turbulence and sometimes the immediate chaos, of social work practice and front-line teams. This is the antithesis of the inquiry and blame culture which often characterizes media and political responses to a tragic event (see Butler and Drakeford 2003; Jones 2003; Stanley and Manthorpe 2004 for critical comments on formal inquiries and reviews).

'Being human' also means not hiding one's own distress and upset, although this should be controlled and not overwhelming for others. However, it does appropriately present the manager (or social worker) as human and emotionally in touch. 'Being human' means celebrating and acknowledging, and it should not be too difficult within social work agencies to find reasons to give recognition to, and to say 'thank you' and 'well done', to colleagues.

'Keeping informed' is about knowing what is happening and what it is really like in day-to-day practice for service users and front-line workers and teams. One of the findings of the Laming Report (2003) (the Victoria Climbié Inquiry) was how out of touch senior managers seemed to be about what was happening in front-line teams and their lack of knowledge about the competence and behaviours of team managers.

There would be (and have been) concerns if social workers were not seeking for themselves a view and understanding of what was happening to a child within a family, or an older person who was isolated and alone. The same expectations and requirements, about being in touch and directly seeing and experiencing, should apply to managers, including senior managers, even if this causes some tensions within line management structures.

'Being honest' is about not hiding from reality or distorting the presentation of reality. For example, the money which has been made available for social care does not stretch to meeting all the aspirations (which are usually very modest and limited) or needs of children, or disabled and older people, who need assistance. A whole raft of jargon has been invented, some of it within government guidance – such as 'eligibility criteria' or 'targeting' – to describe what is in essence *not* providing the assistance some people need and which would enhance their lives. This information needs to be placed in the public arena and needs to be made explicit, with descriptions of unmet need and talk of 'rationing' assistance.

'Being honest' is also about recognizing failure and poor performance and then setting out to tackle it, but not primarily by retreating behind a wall of blame. And when action has to be taken to address poor individual performance it can still be tackled in a way which does not duck the issue and the management responsibility, but which still recognizes people's contribution and strengths as well as where they have been weak or wrong (even when the outcome is disciplinary action, including dismissal).

'Being honest' is also about recalling one's own past performance, fears and hesitancies (which is why there should be a benefit from managers having also been practitioners), such as the uncertainties, ambivalence and the sense of 'feeling lost' when confronted, especially when less experienced, with threatening and violent parents, very challenging adolescents, or the confusion and disturbance of someone experiencing a severe mental health or personal life-changing crisis.

'Managing role conflicts and tensions' arises where one action competes and conflicts with another. For example, having to make cuts in services (while being explicit about the impact this will have) does not lie at all easily with continuing (at least in a public arena) to advocate against such cuts. This is why it is sometimes necessary to create, and to defer to, another party (such as, in this example, a user-led collective advocacy organization) to continue to challenge the actions being taken (but then to ensure that the other party's funding still remains secure and their reputation is not undermined through seeking to discredit their argument).

Such apparent conflicts frequently arise for social workers. For example, they may need to take action through the courts to protect children and yet also have a need to stay close to and maintain the trust of the parents. Or they may need to call on a separate resource to help a disabled person to represent themselves in discussion with the social worker. If social workers can and are expected to manage these role tensions, then it is logical to expect them to retain these skills as they move into organizational management roles.

Successful, high-performing authorities, with good staff morale, have managers who do behave like this (see Social Services Inspectorate/Audit Commission undated), and this is also reflected in commercial business where successful companies have been found to be those who are clear about their goals, stay focused and create and sustain a workforce which is confident, competent and motivated to deliver (see e.g. Collins 2001).

And as Collins (2006: 26) noted:

Consistency distinguishes the truly great – consistent intensity of effort ... consistency with core values, consistency over time. Enduring great institutions practice the principles of Preserve Core Values and Stimulate Progress, separating core values and fundamental purpose (which should never change) from mere operating principles, cultural norms and business strategy (which endlessly adapt to a changing world).

There is here again a focus on values – Collins is writing about what he called the 'social sectors' but also draws on his research on commercial sectors, for whom he has the same message.

Social work and management: some tips

Towards the beginning of this chapter it was noted that social workers are themselves managers. Managing is not only about 'managing down', although this is how management is seen when it is something done to others by people with more formal status positions, seniority and power within organizations. It is also about 'managing in, out and up'.

'Managing in' is about managing the self, including one's own emotions, behaviour and presentation. How one is perceived by others (inspiring, confident, enthusiastic, committed or careless, lazy, disrespectful, selfish), and how one feels about oneself (confident, energized, stimulated or panicky, fed up, confused) impacts on one's ability to perform and how others perceive that performance. This is not exclusively about business or line management; it is about life generally and it is certainly about being a social worker.

'Managing out' is about relationships with, and responses to, service users, team colleagues and partners in other agencies and in the community more generally. It is about building and sustaining credibility and respect, about constructive joint working, and about having influence and a positive (or negative!) impact.

'Managing up' is about remembering that line managers can be influenced and shaped as well as be influencing and shaping. For example, when a manager comes to meet with a front-line team, how does the team decide to play it?

- Option one: offload immediately and continuously about all the pressures experienced by the team, about the bureaucracy and about the lack of resources, with the manager more and more cornered and reacting defensively.

- Option two: balance the presentation by initially talking about the team's achievements, giving recognition to others if appropriate, and then raising the issues which are of concern, with the manager by then already engaged in the discussion and more likely to be more open.

However, it is not only when a manager initiates contact with a team that team members can have an impact. This may not work with all managers, but initiating contact with managers to share information, to make proposals or to raise concerns and issues is also a part of 'managing up'.

Principles and pragmatism

But what about when the political or organizational context is in considerable opposition to the value base of social work? There will and should always be bottom lines which should not be crossed when actions run totally counter to professional and personal values. A recent example is the government's policy intention of removing children from 'failed' asylum seekers and refugees as a deterrent to parents seeking to remain within the UK. In addition to professional (e.g. through the British Association of Social Workers) and managerial (e.g. through the Associations of Directors of Children's Services and Adult Social Services) opposition to this policy, personal and professional values and commitments should not allow social workers or managers to take action to remove children from asylum seekers. If then challenged by their employing organizations it may be necessary to refer back to the GSCC's codes for employers and for social workers and, if required, to fight it out (whatever the consequence).

A similar stance might be appropriate if an agency, for example, introduced a standard overriding policy which set a financial limit on assistance for disabled or older people living in the community, matched against a threshold of the cost of residential or nursing home care. This is likely to run counter to the Human Rights Act principles regarding a right to family life.

But what about when a situation is less clear cut?

A particular thorny experience for social workers and managers is the heavy rationing of services, because the money available does not meet all the needs being identified. The consequence is people being left with a poorer quality of life, and potentially at a continuing high level of danger and stress.

When within local authorities there were committees meeting in public, the senior managers could report their concerns to the committee in the public arena where there would be open political debate. The personal consequences of heavy rationing then became a public and political issue both locally and nationally. Currently however, one-party state cabinet government within local authorities (with the national government demanding that local councils are run by 'cabinets', where decisions are taken by a small group of senior councillors, usually from one political party, rather than through open debate) means that decisions are often taken outside the public arena and the information and advice provided to leading politicians within the cabinet is unseen, and the dialogue, debate and disagreements never heard, by others. How this state of affairs is handled differs from context to context and authority to authority. The commitment to transparency and openness, and the acceptance and toleration of senior managers reporting and speaking in public or across political groups, also varies.

This is where managers (and social workers) need to be politically adept and pragmatic. It does not mean caving in or giving up. It does mean supporting and creating alliances with others (including user-controlled organizations) who may be able to make the public comments which cannot directly be made by the managers. It also means collectively (as social workers and as managers) joining together to create shared voices (through trade union, professional and managerial associations) while accepting that they may not always be in unison.

Conclusion

This chapter has been about the feasibility and desirability of building shared agendas and ambitions between practice and management, between social workers and social work and social care managers. Each role (practitioner and manager) holds its own stresses, tensions and conflicts. Each role-holder is limited and restricted by the political, organizational and resource contexts in which they work. But holding on to a shared value base and – whether as a social worker or manager – recognizing and using the skills and competencies which are a part of good social work, provides the opportunity to build and champion shared agendas alongside and shaped by service users.

References

Abdela, L. (1991) *Breaking Through the Glass Ceiling.* London: Metropolitan Authorities Recruitment Agency.

Abdela, L. (1995) *Do It! Walk the Talk.* London: Metropolitan Authorities Recruitment Agency.

Adair, J. (2006) *Leadership and Motivation.* London: Kogan Page.

Bamford, T. (1990) *The Future of Social Work.* Basingstoke: Macmillan.

Barclay Report (1982) *Social Workers: Their Roles and Tasks.* London: Bedford Square Press.

Biestek, F. (1961) *The Casework Relationship.* London: Unwin.

BIOSS (Brunel Institute of Organisations and Social Studies)(1974) *Social Services Departments: Developing Patterns of Work and Organisation.* London: Heinemann.

BIOSS (Brunel Institute of Organisations and Social Studies) (1980) *Organising Social Services Departments.* Heinemann.

British Association of Social Workers (1977) *The Social Work Task.* Birmingham: BASW.

Burns, J. (1978) *Leadership.* New York: Harper & Row.

Butler, I. and Drakeford, M. (2003) *Scandal, Social Policy and Social Welfare.* Bristol: Policy Press.

Butt, H. and Palmer, B. (1985) *Value For Money in the Public Sector.* Oxford: Blackwell.

Collins, J. (2001) *Good To Great.* London: Random House.

Collins, J. (2006) *Good To Great and the Social Sector.* London: Random House.

Coulshed, V., Mullender, A., Jones, D.N. and Thompson, N. (2006) *Management in Social Work.* Basingstoke: Palgrave Macmillan.

Department for Education and Skills (2003) *Every Child Matters,* Cm 5860. London: The Stationery Office.

Department of Health (1998) *Modernising Social Services: Promoting Independence, Improving Protection, Raising Standards,* Cm 4169. London: The Stationery Office.

Department of Health (2005) *Independence, Well-being and Choice: Our Vision for the Future of Social Care for Adults in England,* Cm 6499. London: The Stationery Office.

Department of Health (2006) *Our Health, Our Care, Our Say: A New Direction for Community Services,* Cm 6737. London: The Stationery Office.

Flood, M. and Pease, B. (2005) Undoing men's privilege and advancing gender equality in public sector institutions, *Policy and Society,* 24(4): 119–38.

Flynn, N. (1990) *Public Sector Management.* Hemel Hempstead: Harvester Wheatsheaf.

Gilroy, P. (2004) *A Personal Perspective on the Future of Social Work and Social Care Services in the UK*. Brighton: Pavilion.

Goleman, D. (1996) *Emotional Intelligence*. London: Bloomsbury.

Goleman, D., Boyatzi, P. and McKee, A. (2002) *The New Leaders: Transforming the Art of Leadership into the Science of Results*. London: Little, Brown.

GSCC (General Social Care Council) (2007) *Roles and Tasks of Social Work in England: A Consultation Paper*. London: GSCC.

Harris, J. (2003) *The Social Work Business*. London: Routledge.

Hartley, J. and Allison, M. (2003) The role of leadership in the modernisation and improvement of public services, in J. Reynolds, J. Henderson, J. Seden, J. Charlesworth and A. Bullman (eds) *The Managing Care Reader*. London: Open University/Routledge.

Holman, B. (1993) *A New Deal for Social Welfare*. Oxford: Lion.

International Federation of Social Workers (2000) *International Definition of Social Work*. International Federation of Social Workers.

Jones, R. (2003) Delayering decisions, *ADSS Inform*: 24–5.

Jordan, B. and Jordan, C. (2000) *Social Work and the Third Way: Tough Love and Social Policy*. London: Sage.

Laming Report (2003) *The Victoria Climbié Inquiry*, Cm 5730. London: The Stationery Office.

Martin, V. and Henderson, E. (2001) *Managing in Health and Social Care*. London: Open University/ Routledge.

Nadler, D. and Tushman, M. (1989) Leadership for organisational change, in A. Mohrman, S. Mohrman, G. Ledford, T. Cummings and E. Lawler (eds) *Large-Scale Organisational Change*. San Francisco: Jossey Bass.

Scottish Executive (2006) *Changing Lives*. Edinburgh: Scottish Executive.

Social Services Inspectorate/Audit Commission (undated) *People Need People: Realising the Potential of People Working in Social Services*. London: Audit Commission.

Stanley, N. and Manthorpe, J. (2004) *The Age of Inquiry: Learning and Blaming in Health and Social Care*. London: Routledge.

Welsh Assembly (2006) *A Strategy for Social Services in Wales Over the Next Decade*. Cardiff: Welsh Assembly.

EXERCISE 1

That 'vision' thing

> Students should think about a social care organization they have recently worked in and relate this to Ray Jones' chapter and the following quote:
>
> > ... with a focus on organizations as organic systems with formal and informal cultures, recognizing that relationships are the medium for much activity, that motivation and morale are key in setting and delivering a vision and direction, with learning and feeding back being central to performance, and with an emphasis on leadership ...
>
> - Does the organization you work(ed) in have a shared vision of its work?
> - Was that vision known to all the staff/users?
> - How was it developed?
> - How much were staff and users encouraged to contribute to creating the 'aims' and 'objectives' of the organization?

 EXERCISE 2

What makes a good and effective manager?

> Students should be asked to make a list of the attributes and qualities they think make a good and effective manager and compare them with their own experiences of being managed.
>
> - Can this list be put in a coherent order?
> - On what basis have you compiled your list?
> - What has been your actual experience and how does the management you have experienced measure against the 'ideal'?

 EXERCISE 3

Visible managers?

> Students should read the following quote from p. 154 and match it to their experience of managers when the going gets tough:

It also means being 'out there' when the going gets tough and when, as is bound to happen from time to time, there is a dramatic event such as a child being seriously injured or dying, or a disabled or older person being stranded without the essential assistance they require.

Organizations often speak about a 'no blame culture' and being a 'learning organization'. For managers this should mean being close to front-line staff and being recognized as understanding the realities, including the turbulence and sometimes the immediate chaos, of social work practice and front-line teams.

- When things have been difficult or very stressful, how 'senior' has been the 'visible' support from managers?
- How 'high' up the hierarchy has the support been provided?
- What forms has this support taken?

 EXERCISE 4

Building alliances?

On page 159 Ray Jones talks about how decisions concerning funding and resources are often made 'behind closed doors':

> It does mean supporting and creating alliances with others (including user-controlled organizations) who may be able to make the public comments which cannot directly be made by the managers. It also means collectively (as social workers and as managers) joining together to create shared voices ...

Students should think about this quote and discuss it, bearing in mind that Jones is suggesting (in part) that workers in social care should be more proactive and creative in their alliances.

- Can you think of any active alliances in your organization where service users and workers work collectively for better resources?
- Is it appropriate to be asking that front-line workers and service users create the means of having their views and voices heard? If so, what might these means be?
- What do you think are the challenges and obstacles you face in forming better alliances with service users?

Students should refer to Chapter 6 by Peter Beresford and to the 'Shaping Our Lives' website (www.shapingourlives.org.uk) and consider evidence, ideas, methods and preconditions for collaborations with service users.

chapter **eleven**

ANTI-SOCIAL CARE: OCCUPATIONAL DEPRIVATION AND OLDER PEOPLE IN RESIDENTIAL CARE

Joan Healey

In this chapter I will be exploring some critical issues associated with social care and our value base, in specific relation to the occupational deprivation of vast numbers of older people in society today. I will do this in the context of my own profession – occupational therapy – but must emphasize that the concepts and issues explored are applicable to all social care contexts, as ageism and oppressive practice are apparent everywhere. However, the notion of enforced 'inactivity' – occupational deprivation – raises issues of human rights and, consequently, managers and practitioners in social care settings must face the dilemmas of developing services for an emerging older population. There is a desperate need to look at how we use public/private and service user partnerships and how we create services, resources and opportunities which embrace innovative practice. One day, if we are lucky, we will all be old. None of us are immune to the ageing process, and the opportunity to remain creative and active is an essential human right.

As far back as 1981 Peter Townsend was discussing the effects of 'enforced dependence' on older people in residential care. In his definitive study, he outlined how residential care was organized around 'caring for' and 'helping' residents at the expense of their self-determination:

> The routine of residential homes, made necessary by small staffs and economical administration and committed to an ideology of 'care and attention' rather than the encouragement of self help and self management, seems to deprive many residents of the opportunity if not the incentive to occupy themselves and even of the means of communication.
>
> (p. 20)

Since then there has been little evidence of a fundamental shift in this style of service provision towards user empowerment, partnership and collaborating with users. What does this say about how we as a society view and value the older person?

There have also been major developments in pension provision in western society which have created another group of 'older people' whose very distinction seems to be their affluence and ability to remain active and engaged in society. While activity is lauded as a key ingredient of healthy ageing in wider western society, in social care it has been relegated to a luxury, coming at the bottom of the list after caring and domestic procedures.

The role of occupation in healthy living

As a profession, occupational therapy is repositioning itself away from medical model concepts of occupation and activity as a means to enhancing people's function after illness or trauma, and is moving more towards analysing and enabling groups and communities to engage in meaningful occupation as a right of self-expression and human dignity (Kronenberg *et al.* 2005). The emergence of occupational science as an academic discipline has added much needed intellectual debate and research-based evidence to highlight the pivotal role that 'doing' plays in our lives in society (Wilcock 1999; Whiteford 2000; Yerxa 2000). If we as a profession value occupation as a life-enhancing and engaging component of our interactions with the world, then we must also redefine our relationships with service users and our spheres of work to address the consequences of this. Older people's place in society, like anyone else's, is often defined by what they do. If they are not allowed to do anything, if they are occupationally deprived, then they are placed outside of and excluded from society. Whiteford (2000: 200) defines occupational deprivation as 'in essence, a state in which a person or a group of people are unable to do what is necessary and meaningful in their lives due to external restrictions'.

Ageing in western society

Ageing is the subject of various cultural discourses today, usually focused around the premise that to display signs of ageing is to display signs of failure. '*Anti-ageing*' is the buzzword of the fashion, cosmetics and lifestyle industries in our media-dominated society. *Positive ageing* is the mantra of our health and social care services. The concept of bipolar ageism has been discussed by various sociologists who point out that the 'positive' images only seek to copy the values held as important in youth – keeping active and keeping productive – and that these stereotypes do not allocate any value to ageing in itself (Cole 1992; Blaikie 1999; Bytheway 2000; McHugh 2003). One cannot win either way – the very concept of the healthy, active ageing person only serves to highlight the mirror image of the dependent person in physical decline that they are keeping at bay by maintaining their youth.

Just as with much health promotion literature and policy, the emphasis in western societies is now on the responsibility being with the individual to maintain their health into old age (Higgs and Gilleard 2006; Rudman 2006): it is our responsibility to make sure that we are financially secure and fit when we reach retirement. If we are not then the reverse is often assumed – it is our own fault, it is because of something we have done or failed to do (Rudman 2006). If this is the case, then how different is the residential care home from the workhouse of the nineteenth century and what is the impact of this on the person who is forced to go into residential care because of illness or lack of social support (Higgs and Gilleard 2006)?

Our very definitions of old age are changing. Recent policy in the UK has started to identify older age beginning at 50 – which given longer life expectancies means that some of us can look forward to being 'old' for almost half of our lives. At the same time, this period of 'older age' has become further divided, firstly into the now accepted stage of the Third Age (Laslett 1989), which seems to be held to be the time between retirement from paid work and ill-health and physical decline, this latter period then becoming the Fourth Age. The population is ageing and the experience of people who have lived over 50 years on this planet is changing rapidly too. Is the concept of 'older people' really a useful one at all? Can such a diverse group of peoples ever be usefully lumped together as a category when their only connection is the amount of time they have lived? What purpose does it serve?

Living beyond retirement

Because of improvements in health care in the post-war years in western society and the emergence of cohorts of people who have paid into pension funds, the experience of living beyond retirement has changed for a substantial number of people. The new groupings of people who are relatively financially well off and fit have created a new category of society member, not dependent on work to support them, not dependent on the state, but independently resourced and focused. The image of the fit and active 60-year-old, travelling the world, taking on new hobbies, with a wide social circle well beyond family, is a cultural reference point which our society seems to be still coming to terms with. In a global economy, what role do such people have other than as another consumer group to be exploited? Compare this to a 100 years ago in this society and to other cultures before the onset of global capitalism, where an older person's role was still defined by their work and family, employment and income, or family caring tasks and support. As global capitalism makes its mark on all cultures, roles and responsibilities are changed, and old age is no longer just defined by cultural norms.

Older age and human rights

If we see occupation as one of the key ways in which we interact with our world (Yerxa 2000), then having the right to this, having access to choice about what we do and where and when we do it, is a fundamental human right. When Townsend revisited his 1981 study in 2006 he advocated using the human rights framework as a means to changing policy and services for older people for the better. He specifically looks at the European Social Chapter as a possible vehicle for demanding change. He notes, as do others (Thompson and Thompson 2001) that while service user involvement in some areas has developed considerably, notably among adult mental health service users, it has not developed anywhere near as rapidly among older people's services. Solutions to social exclusion, although very high on the current government agenda in Britain, are targeted at younger age groups and rarely applied to older people.

In spite of government initiatives and policy since the NHS Plan (Department of Health 2000) and the National Service Framework (Department of Health 2001), staff in the health service still talk of services entitled 'care of the elderly' or 'geriatric medicine'. There are still some fundamental attitudinal discrepancies evident in types of service provision and the language used to describe it. These belie an ethical assumption which relates back to the concepts discussed earlier about good and bad ageing. Ageing is good when it can't be seen or when it is minimal ageing, but when it means illness or loss of abilities then ageing is bad because it means a person is less than independent and therefore in need of support from society (Rudman 2006), and will have a cost to the Exchequer.

In today's western society of advanced consumer ideals, dependence is bad. Feminist ethics have challenged this assumption for many years (Lloyd 2004) and ask us to think about concepts of co-dependence and interdependence: we may at any time in our lives experience periods when we are vulnerable and dependent on other people, and this is a natural part of life experience, not one that is solely attached to age or ability/ disability. Viewing dependence like this would de-stigmatize it and disassociate it from specific groups of marginalized people.

Occupation, integration and involvement

If occupation is viewed as a crucial element of 'positive' ageing, how can we promote and value it so highly for one group of older people, and positively deny it to another? In occupational therapy and occupational science literature, the effects of occupational deprivation among sections of the population are being documented. Mozley (2001) looked at the effects of occupation on care home residents' mental health and found that opportunities for occupation and pleasure had a direct influence on people's mood states and survival rates.

In literature from national governments to the World Health Organization (WHO), occupation and activity play an important role in definitions concerning health. Indeed, engaging in leisure activities and social participation are an integral component of the WHO's classification of function. What is it then about the environments and culture of residential care homes which fosters this occupational deprivation and isolation from society as whole? Why are residential homes for older people so often isolated from the community around them? Why do so many residents remain within the four walls of residential homes once they move in? Why is the link with the wider community non-existent? An attitudinal culture about older people as 'past it' or having nothing to offer to society pervades the very design of these buildings.

Organization and provision of residential care

For part of the answer to these questions we need to look at the provision of residential care itself. Although it is categorized as 'social' care, much of it is now provided by the private sector and big business. In 2004, residential care was valued at £10.2 billion, the private sector accounting for £6.9 billion of this (Drakeford 2006). 'Care' is paid for either from individual savings, including sales of homes, or by the local authority – in fact, in 2004, 61 per cent of residents were paid for by local authorities (Drakeford 2006). Currently the market for residential care provision is dominated by a few very large financial businesses that have multi-million pound turnovers. The profit margins are the subject of much competition. Workers in care homes are low-paid and under-skilled and have poor conditions of service compared to similar public service provision. Care homes are currently an area of employment attracting workers from across Europe and it is not unusual for residential homes to lose much of their workforce when a supermarket opens in the area and offers better pay and conditions than residential care work. It is a service that needs to make its shareholders rich and so pays low wages. Quality of care is implicitly bound by and within these restrictions.

Government policy on improving services for older people abounds and there is recognition in this policy that massive changes need to be made to social care for older people generally. The Department of Health in 2005 set out its aims to help older people by ensuring more control, more choice, more chance to do everyday things and improved quality support and protection. The Wanless Report (2006) looked at the future of care for older people as we anticipate an increase of two-thirds in the numbers of people age 85 and over by the year 2026 compared with an overall increase in population of just 10 per cent. One of the Report's findings was that too many people who could have been supported at home had been admitted to residential care *against their wishes* (Media briefing, March 2006). Is residential care a punishment for not keeping young, healthy and financially solvent?

Conclusion

In 'life' as occupational beings we all set ourselves tasks and goals for the day, the week, the year, and we make choices about what, when and how we do things. Most people have to conform to certain rules and routines in order to function in society, but within that we still make decisions for ourselves about the smallest little things, from whether to have a biscuit with our cup of tea, to much more important things such as who we spend time with. We are all constrained by resources and accessibility, but someone in residential care may have even the smallest opportunity for choice taken from them. A resident of a care home has very little chance to exercise any control over their environment or their routine – things which make us individuals and allow us to express our sense of self and who we are. By depriving older people in residential care of the ability to engage in meaningful occupation we are depriving them of the right to self-expression and a sense of identity. Occupation also has another role in dividing up our day into routines, giving it structure, variety and pattern that highlights our relationship with the world (Whiteford 2000). Without this, time becomes a blank space and our relationship with it is lost – days become one and the same, weeks and seasons run into one, and we can lose a sense of life as it is lived or was lived.

Article 27 in the United Nations Declaration of Human Rights states that everyone has the right to participate in the cultural life of the community and to enjoy the arts, yet how many people in residential care are able to exercise this right? Is providing an activity organizer for two sessions a week really addressing people's needs or is it merely complying with minimum standards and ticking a box in the inspectorate's audit? Without the means to express individuality in what we do, we live only half a life. As a society we extol the virtues of keeping active and engaged in society while wilfully denying it to certain groups of people – prisoners, refugees, homeless people and older people in residential care. The tacit presumption of blame is readily apparent in that grouping.

Changes in health and longevity, financial resources and pensions mean that 'old age' as we knew it even 20 years ago is no longer a useful concept. Redesigning services for older people without the financial resources and flexibility for them to buy and choose their own living arrangements will always reflect the values of the society in which we live. Being beyond working age conveys no value. If governments really want to change cultures in service provision for older people then service users must be centrally involved in the architecture of this transformation.

References

Blaikie, A. (1999) *Ageing and Popular Culture.* Cambridge: Cambridge University Press.

Bytheway, B. (2000) Youthfulness and agelessness: a comment, *Ageing and Society*, 20: 781–9.

Cole, T.R. (1992) *The Journey of Life: A Cultural History of Ageing in America.* Cambridge: Cambridge University Press.

Department of Health (2000) *NHS Plan: A Plan for Investment, a Plan for Reform*. London: The Stationery Office.

Department of Health (2001) *National Service Framework for Older People*. London: The Stationery Office.

Department of Health (2005) *Independence, Well-being and Choice*. London: The Stationery Office.

Drakeford, M. (2006) Ownership, regulation and public interest: the case of residential care for older people, *Critical Social Policy*, 26(4): 932–44.

Higgs, P. and Gilleard, C. (2006) Departing the margins: social class and later life in a second modernity, *Journal of Sociology*, 42(3): 219–41.

Kronenberg, F., Aldago, A. and Pollard, N. (2005) *Occupational Therapy Without Borders*. Edinburgh: Churchill Livingstone.

Laslett, P. (1989) *A Fresh Map of Life*. London: Weidenfield & Nicholson.

Lloyd, L. (2004) Mortality and morality: ageing and the ethics of care, *Ageing and Society*, 24: 235–56.

McHugh, K. (2003) Three faces of ageism: society, image and place, *Ageing and Society*, 23: 165–85.

Mozley, C. (2001) Exploring connections between occupation and mental health in care homes for older people, *Journal of Occupational Science*, 8(3): 14–19.

Rudman, D. (2006) Shaping the active, autonomous and responsible modern retiree: an analysis of discursive technologies and their links in the neo-liberal political rationality, *Ageing and Society*, 26: 181–201.

Thompson, N. and Thompson, S. (2001) Empowering older people, *Journal of Social Work*, 1(1): 61–76.

Townsend, P. (1981) The structured dependency of the elderly: a creation of social policy in the twentieth century, *Ageing and Society*, 1(1): 5–28.

Wanless, D. (2006) *Securing Good Care for Older People: Taking a Long-term View*. London: King's Fund.

Whiteford, G. (2000) Occupational deprivation: a global challenge in the new millenium, *British Journal of Occupational Therapy*, 63(5): 200–5.

Wilcock, A. (1999) Reflections on doing, being and becoming, *Australian Journal of Occupational Therapy*, 46: 1–11.

Yerxa, E. (2000) Confessions of an occupational therapist who became a detective, *British Journal of Occupational Therapy*, 63(5): 192–8.

EXERCISE 1

What do you want to be when you grow up?

Write a list of all the things you do in a typical day, starting from when you get up through to when you go to sleep at night. Apart from the things you have to do in order to live, such as eat, dress, walk etc., think about how much of your time you spend doing things you *choose* to do. Ask yourself the following questions:

- How much do you do with other people and how much do you do alone?
- What are the most important things to you?
- What roles do you fulfil?
- How many different roles do you have in a day (e.g. parent, sister, brother, partner, aunt, uncle, student, teacher, role model)?
- Now imagine yourself at 80. How many roles do you have now? How many things do you still want to do? What roles would you still hope to be playing? How important is it to be able to choose what you want to do?

The exercise is an attempt to highlight the extent of 'unoccupation' in later life and how we would not necessarily choose to live this way.

 EXERCISE 2

Who do you know who is old?

- Outside your immediate family, how many friends over 70 do you have?
- Who are they?
- How did you get to know them?
- Tell your group about their personality, likes and dislikes.
- How long have you known them?

EXERCISE 3

How are older people valued around the world?

Create a list of culturally different countries from around the world. Ask the students to pick a country out of a hat and then research the extent to which older people are valued in that country.

- Have older people ever been valued in that society?
- What provisions are there for older people?
- What is the state pension (and the minimum wage)?
- In what part(s) of the world are older people valued the most?

INDEX